I0055626

MEDICAL COMMUNICATION

From Theoretical Model to Practical Exploration

MEDICAL COMMUNICATION
From Theoretical Model to Practical Exploration

Tao Wang
Shanghai East Hospital,
Tongji University School of Medicine, China

Zhongqing Xu
Tongren Hospital,
Shanghai Jiao Tong University School of Medicine, China

Yi Mou
School of Media and Communication,
Shanghai Jiao Tong University, China

W World Century

Published by

World Century Publishing Corporation

27 Warren Street, Suite 401-402, Hackensack, NJ 07601, USA

Library of Congress Control Number: 2020940138

British Library Cataloguing-in-Publication Data
A catalogue record for this book is available from the British Library.

《医学传播学：从理论模型到实践探索》
Originally published in Chinese by Shanghai Scientific & Technological Education Publishing House Co., Ltd.
Copyright © 2019 by Wang Tao, Mou Yi, Xu Zhongqing.
English translation rights arranged with Shanghai Scientific & Technological Education Publishing House Co., Ltd.

MEDICAL COMMUNICATION
From Theoretical Model to Practical Exploration

Copyright © 2020 by World Century Publishing Corporation

All rights reserved. This book, or parts thereof, may not be reproduced in any form or by any means, electronic or mechanical, including photocopying, recording or any information storage and retrieval system now known or to be invented, without written permission from the publisher.

For photocopying of material in this volume, please pay a copying fee through the Copyright Clearance Center, Inc., 222 Rosewood Drive, Danvers, MA 01923, USA. In this case permission to photocopy is not required from the publisher.

ISBN 978-1-945552-09-0 (hardcover)
ISBN 978-1-945552-10-6 (ebook for institutions)
ISBN 978-1-945552-11-3 (ebook for individuals)

For any available supplementary material, please visit
https://www.worldscientific.com/worldscibooks/10.1142/U035#t=suppl

Contents

About the Authors

Tao Wang

- Director, Center for Health and Medical Communication, School of Media and Communication, Shanghai Jiao Tong University, China;
- Director, Emergency Management and Disaster Public Opinion Research Center, School of Arts and Media, Tongji University, China;
- Director, Health and Medical Communication Research Center, School of Television Arts, Communication University of Zhejiang, China;
- Executive Director, Disaster Response Branch, Joint Research Center for Health Policy of Shanghai Jiao Tong University and Yale University;
- Executive Deputy Director of Emergency Medicine Department and Director of Emergency Management Office of Shanghai East Hospital, Tongji University School of Medicine, China.

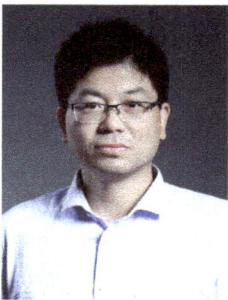

Dr. Wang obtained his undergraduate medical training at the Shanghai Second Medical University, China, and his master's degree in Surgery at Tongji University, China. He has over 20 years of experience working in orthopedic trauma clinic at Shanghai Sixth People's hospital. He has published more than 80 academic papers in leading journals including *The Lancet*. He has won the second prize of China National Science and Technology Progress Award. In 2018 he was invited as a special guest to the Academician Conference of the Chinese Academy of Sciences and Chinese Academy of Engineering.

Zhongqing Xu

- Director, General Practice Department, Tongren Hospital, Shanghai, China;
- Vice Director, General Practice Department, Shanghai Jiao Tong University School of Medicine, China;
- Vice Director, Center for Health and Medical Communication, School of Media and Communication, Shanghai Jiao Tong University, China.

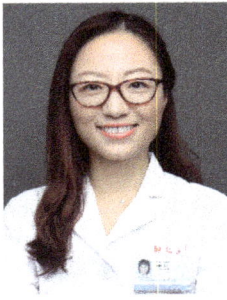

Dr. Xu obtained her undergraduate medical training at the Shanghai Medical University, China, and her master's degree in Internal Medicine at Shanghai Jiao Tong University School of Medicine, China. She was a visiting scholar at the Faculty of Medicine, University of Ottawa in 2017 and studied short-term in HKFCP and RCGP in 2019. She has worked in the emergency department and general practice department of Tongren Hospital for more than 20 years. She has published more than 20 academic papers.

Yi Mou

- Special Researcher, School of Media and Communication, Shanghai Jiao Tong University, China;
- Associate Director, Center for Health and Medical Communication, School of Media and Communication, Shanghai Jiao Tong University, China.

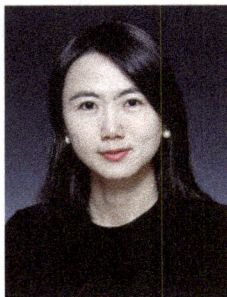

Dr. Mou obtained her Ph.D. in Communication from University of Connecticut in the U.S. Her research interests include new media studies and health communication, such as employing new media tools to achieve health preventive objectives. She has published more than 30 papers in SCI- and SSCI-indexed journals and won several awards from international conferences. She also serves on the editorial boards of five international academic journals.

List of Contributors

Chief Reviewers:

YU Guoming School of Journalism and Communication, Beijing Normal University, China

LI Benqian School of Media and Communication, Shanghai Jiao Tong University, China

Deputy Editors:

WANG Sheng Hangzhou Normal University, China

YUAN Ting Shanghai Sixth People's Hospital, China

Editors: (in alphabetical order)

DAI Yun Tongren Hospital, Shanghai Jiao Tong University School of Medicine, China

GUO Shuzhang Tianjin Third Central Hospital, China

JIA Xiyan Qingbu Branch, Zhongshan Hospital Affiliated to Fudan University, China

JIANG Benran Parkway Health Shanghai, China

JIANG Ping Shanghai Mental Health Center, Shanghai Jiao Tong University School of Medicine, China

SHEN Jian Shuguang Hospital Affiliated to the Shanghai University of Traditional Chinese Medicine, China

XU Hui Shanghai Changning Maternity & Infant Health Hospital, China

XU Lingmin	Qingbu Branch, Zhongshan Hospital Affiliated to Fudan University, China
ZHAO Xiaogang	Shanghai Pulmonary Hospital, China
ZHAO Wensui	Changning District Center for Disease Control and Prevention, Shanghai, China
ZHOU Minjie	Shanghai Sixth People's Hospital East Campus, China

Participants: (in alphabetical order)

FENG Xianzhen	Tongren Hospital, Shanghai Jiao Tong University School of Medicine, China
GAO Hui	Changning District Center for Disease Control and Prevention, Shanghai, China
LU Hong	Tongren Hospital, Shanghai Jiao Tong University School of Medicine, China
WANG Zhean	University of Sydney, Australia
XU Chen	Tongren Hospital, Shanghai Jiao Tong University School of Medicine, China
XU Zhang	Shanghai Jiao Tong University School of Medicine, China
YANG Yinying	Qingbu Branch, Zhongshan Hospital Affiliated to Fudan University, China
ZHANG Lin	School of Media and Communication, Shanghai Jiao Tong University, China

Part I
Generality

Chapter 1

Definition and Characteristics of Medical Communication

For thousands of years, people have gradually accumulated a wealth of medical knowledge in the battle against diseases and have spread the knowledge constantly in different ways. The medical knowledge has gradually developed into different medical systems. More than 2000 years ago, the ancient Greek physician, Hippocrates, the father of modern medicine, issued an oath that *"in every house where I come I will enter only for the good of my patients, keeping myself far from all intentional ill-doing and all seduction and especially from the pleasures of love with women or men, be they free or slaves"*. In Chinese history, the creation of five-animal boxing by the famous doctor in Han dynasty, Hua Tuo, and the popularization of Tusu wine by Sun Simiao, who is respected as the king of medicine, demonstrated the superb medical skills and effective means of dissemination of medical knowledge in the ancient China. Meanwhile, the ancients attached great importance to health education in the medical field. *Huang Di Nei Jing*, the first medical classic in the history of the Warring States period in China, stated: *"The best doctor prevents illness, the better attends to impending sickness and the inferior treats existing illness."* What the sentence means is similar to the concept of disease prevention in modern medicine. It points out that it is more important to prevent diseases than to treat existing diseases and the subject of both treating diseases and preventing diseases is the doctor. Today in the age of communication technology explosion, on the one hand, we are in the age of information explosion, wandering among all kinds of unevenly sourced information. Neither does all medical information come from professional medical staff nor is all medical information true and reliable. On the other hand, the scientific literacy of citizens has not yet reached a high standard. According to the results of the Ninth China Citizens' Scientific Quality Survey released by the China Association for Science and Technology in 2016, the proportion of citizens with science literacy in China is 6.2%. Although there has been a steady improvement compared with the past, compared with western developed countries, there is still a considerable gap, which means that at present in China, the vast majority of citizens do not yet have good scientific literacy. These reasons make it difficult for the citizens to effectively identify correct and useful medical knowledge from today's explosive information flow. Citizens are more likely to be misled by fake news or misinformation, resulting in serious consequences. In recent years, the exposure of fake doctors such as Zhang Wuben and Liu Hongbin, as well as misdiagnosis caused by wrong information are all shown as typical cases. Therefore, in the field of medical communication, citizens generally call for the appearance of "professional team" (medical communication by professional medical personnel). At the same time, the communication practice of medical science popularization by medical staff also urgently needs the guidance of theory.

As a kind of practical activity, medical communication has a long history, but its emergence as an academic field has only recently begun. Medical communication originated from various disciplines such as medicine, history of science, philosophy of science, and communication, and has gradually formed its independent discipline system. We will introduce the definition of medical communication and distinguish its relationship with medical science popularization, health communication, and general science communication one by one. Meanwhile, the characteristics of medical communication will also be proposed.

1. Definition of medical communication

Medical science communication, also called medical communication for short, is about the spread of medical science. Medical communication is a crosscutting field emerging from the medicine and communication, having a close relationship with traditional science popularization. According to American scholars Stephen W. Littlejohn and Karen A. Foss, science communication can be seen as an interdisciplinary meta-field on the branch of discipline. Undoubtedly, medical communication is a very important part of this meta-domain. At the same time, medical communication focuses on the medical personnel engaged in communication and therefore tends towards medicine in terms of subject affiliation.

According to the most basic "5W" model of communication, medical communication contains the following elements:

First, **who** to spread?

Medical communication, as a branch of science communication, emphasizes the authority and scientific facts of information source. Therefore, the transmitter of medical communication must be professional medical staff, such as the medical workers in the front line including doctors, nurses and medical technicians, formal medical institutions with medical qualifications, and medical graduates with high medical literacy. Medical undergraduates cannot be considered as separate transmitters because their medical knowledge is not comprehensive. This is also consistent with the fact that science popularization is usually dominated by frontline scientists.

Communicator is the cornerstone of all science communication. Communicator deviation will bring lessons to the communication abound. The "Zhang Wuben" incident is a typical case. Zhang Wuben claimed himself to be the "first person in Chinese medicine diet." His published book *Eating Back to Eat Out of the Disease* has aroused widespread concern in the society. Especially in February 2010, after being a guest of Hunan Satellite TV's "Bai Ke Quan Shuo," its popularity increased rapidly. Zhang Wuben became the so-called "Traditional Chinese Medicine Master" throughout the country. He proclaimed the "Mung bean cures all diseases" rule, which even caused the price of mung beans to soar in the market. He disseminated his concepts very well. Later, some media reported that Zhang Wuben was suspected of academic fraud. His exaggerated concept of dietetic therapy was also questioned by experts. Everyone despised "Master Zhang" at that time. Hunan TV's show was also stopped on June 7, 2010. The source of the farce is that Zhang Wuben is not a medical professional as he proclaimed. He was a laid-off worker from a textile factory. He became the so-called "the first batch of senior nutrition experts of the Ministry of Health", even "the first person of traditional Chinese medicine diet therapy" through marketing. His various health concepts, including the "mung bean cures all diseases", do not have a basic medical foundation. He has no basic medical knowledge. A "master" with no professional skills spread his concepts everywhere and caused widespread misdirection and bad impact on the public. It can be seen that the influence of subject deviation on the impact of communication can be devastating. When making medical communication, we must ensure the professionalism of the subject. The subject of communication is the basis of the communication.

Some people may question why medical communication must be based on professional medical staff and why the spread of medical or health knowledge by other personnel cannot be included in the scope of medical communication. Medicine is defined as the subject of dealing with various diseases or lesions of the human body by scientific or technical methods. It is an applied discipline of biology, an advanced science in the treatment of human diseases from anatomical and molecular genetic aspects and a system from prevention to treatment of diseases. The areas of medicine include basic medicine, clinical medicine, forensic science, laboratory medicine, preventive medicine, health medicine, rehabilitation medicine, and so forth. Objects of scientific research can be natural or other related fields. Therefore, a certain degree of deviation is allowed. However, the definition of medicine indicates that medicine is a vital area focused on research and dealing with body illness. Any deviation is not allowable during any therapy, otherwise the right to health even to life may be irreparably hurt. As we all know, a medical student has to go through a systematic and long theoretical study, a considerable period of internship and practice, finally to pass the theoretical and practical examination to be accepted as a real doctor. The training of nurses is also similar. They all take a long period. In the long term, through continuous theoretical and practical learning, medical personnel can grasp the necessary medical knowledge and skills, which cannot be replaced by nonprofessional medical personnel's internet search. Medical communication faces the ordinary public. The right of citizens to live and to be healthy is indispensable. If the communicator does not have the necessary medical knowledge, what he disseminates to people is likely to be wrong or even harmful, which may cause immeasurable danger. This is why we must position the communicator of medical communication to professional medical staff. Only professionally trained medical staff can ensure the reliability and authenticity of the communication content so as to minimize the possibility of incorrect medical knowledge dissemination.

In the past, professional medical staff rarely participated in health knowledge popularization or medical communication. The motivation of professional medical staff to disseminate medical knowledge was often based on personal enthusiasm and social responsibility. The lack of relevant incentive mechanism results in the weak sustainability of medical communication. Many medical staff do not pay attention to medical communication and they even think doctors who devote to such jobs are performing unnecessary work. Also, in the assessment of medical personnel at all levels of medical institutions, there is no assessment mechanism for medical communication or medical popularization. Writing ten popular science articles is thought to be less valuable than publishing one journal paper. It is no wonder that Bai Yansong, a member of the national committee of CPPCC and a famous host, appealed that "Medical science popularization work should be included in the business scope of medical workers and medical researchers. Otherwise, it will be difficult to meet the needs of social science." Fortunately, the community has noticed the problem. Shanxi Health and Family Planning Commission has taken the lead to include popular science articles as review criterion in the 2017 annual health care evaluation of senior professional and technical positions. The status of popular science articles has been upgraded to the same as that of academic papers, which encouraged more and more medical staff to invest in health education and medical science popularization. Benefiting from the incentive mechanism, medical staff have more strength in medical science popularization. The establishment and development of medical communication has made the best footnote for the communicator status of professional medical staff.

Second, spread to **whom**?

Broadly speaking, the audience of medical communication includes two parts: the medical and the nonmedical. The internal medical communication is the communication between professionals, usually in the path of the academic community such as journals, conferences, seminars, which will not be covered here. Medical communication pays more attention to the dissemination toward the nonmedical people. Thus, the general public constitutes the object of medical communication. The audience is made up of several groups, which according to the difference in health status, include patients, patients' relatives and friends, susceptible population, and ordinary crowd. Taking diabetes as an example, the audience includes diabetic patients themselves (patients), all relatives and friends of the diabetic patients (relatives and friends of patients), those with diabetes mellitus or body fatness in their families (susceptible population), and people who do not have diabetes or diabetes risk factors (ordinary crowd). Due to the possible genetic effects of diabetes, dietary habits, lifestyle behaviors, and other factors on diabetes, the medical communication to the abovementioned population is indispensable.

Some people may not understand why there are so many objects of medical communication and they may consider it necessary only for patients but not the healthy. However, the reality is more complicated. A person is a unit with social attributes. In the process of resisting disease, it is not enough to rely on the patients to take care of themselves. Help from surrounding groups, including family and friends, becomes more and more necessary. For example, a stroke patient who has a side limb hemiplegia cannot take care of himself even though he has consciousness. Under such circumstances, it is useless to spread the knowledge of how to maintain and care after hemiplegia to the patient himself. These goals cannot be achieved without the help of family members, friends, or nursing staff. Those who care for the patients are the targets of the dissemination of medical knowledge.

There are three levels of prevention: primary, secondary, and tertiary.

Primary prevention, also called cause prevention, is to prevent the onset of illness or injury before disease process begins. Take diabetes as an example. The target of primary prevention is those who are obese, fond of high-calorie diet, lacking exercise, with family history, or other high-risk factors. Primary prevention is the advice about how to eat healthily, how to exercise and control weight to reduce the risk of diabetes.

Secondary prevention, known as "three early" prevention, is the main measure to prevent the progression of the disease and the spread of illness, and to slow down the disease progression. It refers to early diagnosis and prompt treatment of a disease, illness, or injury to prevent more severe problems developing. Also taking diabetes as an example, secondary prevention is for those who may have diabetes. We hope to identify, diagnose, and treat diabetes in the early stages by screening and regular blood glucose measurement.

Tertiary prevention includes interventions that limit disability or enhance rehabilitation from disease, injury, or disability if a patient has elevated diabetes that was not controlled by diet or exercise. Then, the patient may be referred to other specialists to control the blood sugar and avoid complications. Medical communication not only spreads the treatment of diseases but also pays more attention to the prevention of diseases. Thus, everyone should be the target of medical communication since healthy living and behavioral methods are beneficial not only to patients but also to everyone. Long-term persistence may also reduce the incidence of many chronic diseases.

Third, communicate **what**?

Medical communication has a strict choice of the content. Although medical knowledge is all-encompassing and the latest scientific research results are endless, the content suitable for science communication should be strictly controlled. The purpose of medical communication is to disseminate authoritative, accurate, and scientific medical knowledge to the layman, thereby promoting their healthy behavior and maintaining their health. The medical science knowledge that is still inconclusive, is not suitable as content of medical communication. The content of medical communication should be definitive medical science knowledge, including the contents of current medical books, dictionaries, and medical-related national laws. This is the "gold standard" for medical communication.

Content that does not meet the criteria of "conclusive medical science popularization" includes the following:

The research content that is still in the academic debate and not coming into a conclusive stage should be avoided. For example, is genetically modified food safe? Transgene is the transfer of one or several exogenous genes into a specific organism by genetic techniques. Foods produced by using genetically modified organisms as raw materials are genetically modified foods. The safety of genetically modified foods has been controversial since its birth in the United States in the 1980s. Because there are many ingredients in genetically modified foods, which have never been found in traditional foods, countries have developed more stringent safety inspection standards than for general food. Since there is currently no authoritative official conclusion on the safety of genetically modified foods, for the field of medical communication, it is clearly not suitable for promotion and dissemination. We believe that citizens should have the right to know about cutting-edge scientific issues; however, the academic debate is likely to cause public confusion and anxiety and it cannot provide good guidance for healthy behavior, which is far from the purpose of medical communication. Considering that citizens in China are generally at a low level of science literacy, the content of academic contention should be avoided in medical communication.

Recent literature publications and reports, including those published in authoritative medical journals, should be avoided. Just like cutting-edge research in other fields of science, cutting-edge research in medicine is exploratory, which means many of the contents published in the literature have not undergone the check of time and practice. The Han Chunyu incident is a vivid example. In May 2016, Chinese researcher Han Chunyu published the genome editing results of the NgAgo system in the world's top academic journal, *Nature Biotechnology*, and received much attention at home and abroad. Some media even called it the Nobel Prize–winning experiment. However, about 20 Chinese and foreign scholars later questioned that the experiment could not be repeated, which led to the retraction of the paper from the journal. From this point of view, the latest papers published in authoritative academic journals may not stand the test of time. At the same time, the most cutting-edge scientific research has a big gap in the lives of citizens. Therefore, we do not advocate the direct dissemination of medical science popularization content in the academic literature to citizens without the test of time. In September 2018, an Egyptian astrologist together with American scientists completed the study "A homing system targets therapeutic T cells to brain cancer" and published it in the top international journal, *Nature*. The paper claimed that cell therapy has been successfully applied and the technology effectively treats brain tumors. This technology is realized by an immune cell engineered by a so-called "homing system" which passes through the blood–brain barrier and enters the brain tumor entity. The immune cell performs targeted killing of brain tumor cells. In January 2019, an expert from the University of Oxford in the United Kingdom published a positive review of the abovementioned article in another top journal, *The New England Journal of Medicine*, and introduced the technology to the peers enthusiastically. However, this article in *Nature* has been questioned by many medical experts at home and abroad. The editorial office of *Nature* launched a survey and retracted the article on February 20, 2019. On the same day, the editorial office of *The New England Journal of Medicine* retracted the review of the positive significance of the technology. Even papers published in top international journals may be questioned. There is considerable risk in disseminating content that has not been tested by time. This confirms that medical content that has not been precipitated over time is not suitable for direct dissemination to citizens.

We advocate time as the standard for testing truth. Take *in vitro* fertilization (IVF) technology as an example. This technique was first created in 1978 by British professor Robert Edwards. It was not until 2010 that he won the Nobel Prize in Physiology and Medicine for the creation of this technology. A rigorous scientific attitude should be adopted in the field of medical communication similar to that of the Nobel Prize. In the 1980s, when IVF technology was founded at the beginning due to the unpredictability of technology, medical communication is not suitable for the dissemination and popularization of this technology. Today, 40 years later, time has proven that IVF technology is a very mature technology. It brings millions of families with children and vitality that might have been missing. IVF technology is well suited to the content and topic of communication in the field of medical communication. Although advocating time as the standard for testing truth, we must modify the content to keep pace with the times. This is the timeliness of information. Medicine is constantly improving and developing. If the content is still in the book 30 years ago, it is correct but ridiculous. IVF technology at present has much progress compared to 40 years ago, so we should spread the technology based on the current situation. When we do medical communication, the content and technology disseminated should be improved and changed along with the progress in proportion.

The reason why medical communication is so strict about the content of communication is that the rights to live and to be healthy are both the highest rights of everyone. When we were doing medical communication, citizens may accept the communication with a very trusting attitude. There are quite a large number of people who may change their way of life and behavior according to the content of the dissemination, or even change their medical treatment behavior. If the content we spread is not reliable or has not been widely certified, it is likely to be harmful to the health of people or could even threaten their lives, which is likely to hurt citizens' right to be alive and healthy. This is an error that is not allowed for an emerging discipline. Medicine itself is a very rigorous science. Unlike traditional medicine, modern medicine is evidence-based. It requires a large-scale experimental demonstration to prove its effectiveness before it can be gradually promoted. We need to pay attention to this when we plan medical communication. There is a precedent for a treatment that was once considered effective later to be proved ineffective and harmful. We cannot carry out extensive publicity and promotion while the treatment is still in the experimental exploration stage. This is a disrespect for the people and a disrespect for their right to live and to be healthy.

Fourth, through **which** channel?

The channels of medical communication encompass all the ways to transmit. From the face-to-face communication between medical staff, patients, and their families, to the medical communication activities in the community, and to the use of mass media and new media platforms, medical communication uses various communication channels according to the characteristics of different audiences.

In addition to the traditional medical science popularization pathway advocated by the government, today's medical communication makes full use of the advantages of network communication and actively explores the "Internet + science" model. Since 2010, medical health official accounts on Weibo and WeChat have increased rapidly. Take Sina Weibo as an example. Many personal microblogs that are certified as medical professionals, such as "Emergency Department Superwoman Yu" and

"Xiehe Zhang Rongya" have millions of fans, and their published medical information covers a wide range of concerns.

However, Social Media platform has also become a problematic area of medical false information and rumors. A variety of false information under the banner of health has brought harm to the health and property of the people. The wide spread of healthcare information and the dissemination of health knowledge are far from each other. This so-called healthy communication is the rise of packaging for health information content marketing. Many Social Media health care platforms are not supported by professional medical personnel and the quality of communication content cannot be guaranteed, which is contrary to the concept of medical communication. Medical communication through the media platform should be rigorous and deliver accurate medical knowledge, rather than sensational and having profitable effects that are required in the general sense of the media platform. From the position of the communicator of medical communication, the lack of professional medical personnel to support Social Media communication cannot be regarded as a true medical communication, but a pseudo-propagation. Moreover, if there is no regulatory platform, the dissemination of some false medical content is extremely harmful to the public. The Wei Zexi incident illustrated this problem. Wei Zexi (1994–2016) was a 21-year-old Chinese college student who died of cancer after receiving questionable treatment from a hospital that advertised via the search engine. Wei Zexi was diagnosed with synovial sarcoma, a rare form of cancer. When his family were told that there was little hope of treatment in regular tumor hospitals, his family members found a hospital through the online search engine. The hospital claimed to have very advanced bio-immunotherapy that can cure the disease, but it was more expensive. As a result, the family used this unofficially approved bio-immunotherapy and repeatedly sought treatment at the hospital four times. Finally, after running out of all the savings, Wei Zexi died. The general public cannot always identify correct medical information. If the network platform for medical communication cannot be strictly supervised, and there is no support for medical personnel behind the scenes, it may bring a devastating blow to those who cannot identify correct information. Therefore, regardless of the way of communication, the communicator of communication and the content of communication are very important in medical communication. Only by identifying the subject of the communication and the content of the communication can the preparation and reliability of the communication be ensured.

It is worth noticing that communication skill is a very important part in the way of communication. Experienced and skilled doctors are not necessarily good medical communicators. The usual case is that when the experts are having an impassioned speech on the stage, the audience sleep with no attention left. This may be related to communication skills and modes of communication. As mentioned earlier, the dissemination of the fake doctor Zhang Wuben proved to be pseudo-science and pseudo-medicine, but his communication skills can be used for reference. He caught the attention of the people and adopted the appropriate methods and techniques to make his ideas quickly promoted. While as the communicator of medical communication, it is easy for the professional medical staff to forget that the audience of communication are not peers with medical knowledge, but citizens who have no medical foundation. Medical staff often use very professional terminologies when speaking to the public. These contents may benefit their peers, but they may be too difficult for citizens. Therefore, we should use words that are easier to understand and use appropriate metaphors to achieve better results. For example, when we spread cardiovascular and cerebrovascular knowledge to people, we may tell them the illness they need to prevent is "cerebral apoplexy," which could not be understood by public. When it is switched to the word "stroke," it will be easy to understand. For another example, the World Health Organization and our Chinese residents' dietary guidelines require no more than 6 g of salt per day. If we only tell the public that the salt intake cannot exceed 6 g, it is difficult for them to implement. Because when cooking, the public generally do not take the scale to weigh the amount of salt. If the communicator changes the way, telling the public which foods or condiments contain invisible salt, and how to reduce the intake of salt, the effect of such communication will signally increase. Sometimes, it is necessary to have a certain touch on the subject of medical communication. For two books that have the same content, the one named *80 Days to Become Nursing Master* is obviously more acceptable to the general public than the other one named *Family Nursing Knowledge*, since the latter one looks too professional for layman to understand. This can be inferred that proper communication skills have a positive effect on medical communication. Medical communication cares not only about how much reading is available, or how many people pay attention, but also the scientific and normative of medical communication. In order to communicate medical knowledge to a wider population in a common and easy-to-understand way, certain skills are needed.

At present, the new media form has moved toward the Omnimedia and Media Convergence. The various media forms such as radios, TVs, phototapes and videotapes, films, publications, newspapers, magazines, and websites are highly integrated. Due to the high development of the media, we have entered an era of *"everyone communicates, everything is media"*. The channels of communication are extremely prosperous and complicated. These channels are what medical communication needs to study. Meanwhile, we should keep in mind that good-quality content is primarily important.

Fifth, **what** effect does the communication have?

First of all, medical communication is based on scientificity and propagation as two major evaluation indicators.

The aim of medical communication is to popularize medical knowledge to the public. The effect of communication is determined not just by the number of the audience. What is really important includes whether through the communication health indicators are improved, healthy living behaviors are formed, information gaps between doctors and patients are closed, and whether as much as possible the ultimate goal of rational allocation of medical resources is achieved. The first-aid reality-show documentary "Emergency Room Story" filmed by Dragon TV, is the first program to use the fixed camera shooting method, shooting the story of the hospital emergency room in every respect, combining the plot and humanities, with expert interpretation. After the program was broadcasted, many viewers commented "touching" and "understand the doctors." The patient complaint rate in the emergency department of the hospital dropped significantly. This is due to the documentary filming method, which allows the audience to jump out of their medical experience, reexamine the doctor–patient relationship from an objective perspective, realizing mutual trust between people and promoting positive energy. The scientificity is reflected in not only the content but also the topic. The selection of topics is based on time, region, target population or specific public health events, and so on. Take the target population as an example. It is inappropriate to popularize the prevention and treatment of hypertension, hyperlipidemia, and hyperglycemia among primary and middle school students because the students are not at high risk for these diseases. Considering that students are in the stage of growth and their studies are heavy, "How to prevent myopia," "How to get nutrition," "How to prevent obesity," and "How to get through adolescence" are suitable topics of medical communication. As for region, it is very ridiculous to popularize how to save yourself and save others when the tsunami comes in Sichuan Province. Sichuan is a basin with high incidence of earthquakes, while the ocean is much far from there. There have been many earthquakes in history, such as the 2008 Sichuan earthquake, which is still remembered by people. In Sichuan Province, how to save yourself and save others when the earthquake comes is a good topic and the audience is very broad. Take time as an example. The incidence of various diseases varies from time to time. Summer is the season of high incidence of infectious diseases of digestive tract, whereas winter is the season of cardiovascular and cerebrovascular diseases. Medical communication should be timely. If you popularize "heatstroke prevention" in the winter and "prevent frostbite" in the summer, the audience will be rare. When the order is interchanged, it will have a good effect. Taking time as an example, from last winter to this spring, the flu broke out all over the country. At one time, the respiratory, infectious, and pediatric departments of major hospitals were overcrowded. At this time, many medical staff and the media began to give lectures on how to prevent the flu and how to treat the flu. These lectures have received widespread attention. Meanwhile they have played positive roles in the ultimate control of the flu pandemic.

In addition to the scientificity and propagation, effectiveness is the most important evaluation indicator. The effectiveness includes the improvement of the public's health science literacy level, the improvement of relevant health indicators, and the reduction of the incidence of specific diseases through medical communication. The focus of medical communication is not on the number of audiences in a short period of time, but on the fact that after continuous dissemination and popularization, people can really change their behavior and way of life, gradually develop in a healthier direction, and finally achieve the goal of reducing the incidence of disease, mortality, and disability rate, and achieving the goal of promoting the health of the people. The effect of medical communication is similar to the etiological prevention.

2. Relationship between medical communication and medical science popularization

Medical communication is related to but different from medical science popularization. To systematically clarify the differences, we begin with the relationship between them.

Science popularization, as an organized practice, was born in the second half of the 19th century. It uses simple language to report and explain the progress of science and technology to the public. Suffering from world war, western governments generally recognized the importance of raising citizens' support for science and technology. Science popularization is a paradigm that aims to improve public scientific knowledge and scientific literacy. The landmark event at this stage was the establishment of the Royal Science Association in 1799 and the establishment of the Science Promotion Association in 1831. Since the 1950s, popular science in China has been incorporated into the government system. A set of professional science popularization systems has been established from the central cities to the county. It is the state (government), not the public, that is taking advantage of science popularization under this paradigm. Therefore, as the famous scientific historian Liu Huajie said, *"traditional science popularization takes a government position."*

The scientific community at that time (including scientists and relevant decision-makers) believed that the reason why public distrust science is due to an inadequate understanding of science. The United Kingdom and the United States have been conducting scientific mass communication activities under the leadership of the scientific community since the 1980s. During this period, the Royal Society published an important report, *Public Understanding of Science*, in 1985 and stated the Deficit

Model that illustrated that the public did not support science because of the lack of scientific knowledge. In their opinion, if citizens understand science, they will gradually conform to the opinions of scientists and support science. This paradigm is the scientific community position. In the 1990s, the paradigm of Public Understanding of Science was accepted to some extent in China.

A new paradigm of Public Engagement or Participation in Science and Technology (PEST) was created. It is also known as "dialogue mode" or "democratic model". This paradigm argues that the public should be involved in scientific progress, that is, the public participates in setting the scientific agenda as a way of dialogue with the scientific community. The formation of this paradigm brought about the establishment of disciplines in science communication.

We can find the change of the paradigm from traditional medical science popularization to present medical communication. Medical communication is not limited to the dissemination of knowledge about the treatment and the prevention of diseases like the patriotic health campaign launched in the 1950s, which advocated *"hygiene to eliminate the four evils"*. It has more connotations due to the participation of the public. From Figure 1.1, we can roughly understand the relationship between medical communication, medical science popularization, science popularization, and science communication. Science popularization is a kind of social education, which introduces the knowledge of natural science and social science to the general public in a simple way, popularizes the

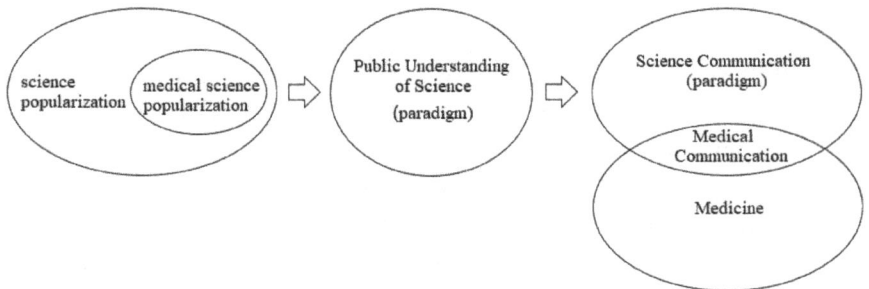

Figure 1.1   Relationship and difference between medical communication and medical science popularization.

application of science and technology, advocates scientific methods, disseminates scientific ideas, and promotes scientific spirit. In the paradigm of science popularization, if the content involved is medical knowledge, it belongs to medical science popularization. Therefore, medical science popularization belongs to science popularization. In the paradigm of science popularization, citizens can understand science and further participate in it, which forms the paradigm of science communication. If the content of science communication is medical knowledge, it is medical communication. Medical communication is the intersection of science communication and medicine. Medical science popularization is not medical communication unless it is understood and effectively participated by the citizens.

The content of medical communication has three levels in details.

First is the talk about "Disease", which is the knowledge of prevention, health care, and rehabilitation of diseases. It is the most understandable and basic level of medical communication. That is the main content of traditional medical science. Taking a very common disease "hypertension" as an example, medical communication needs to be carried out in the following aspects: The first step is the prevention of hypertension mainly for the citizens without high blood pressure and the target population who are likely to have high blood pressure in the future (susceptible population). The content includes which groups of people are susceptible to high blood pressure; how to measure blood pressure in a normal population; how do susceptible populations adjust their diet, exercise, and lifestyle; what are the symptoms of high blood pressure; and other medical content related to hypertension prevention. The second step is the treatment and health care of hypertension mainly for hypertensive (patients) and the relatives and friends of patients. The content includes how hypertensives adjust their diet, exercise, and lifestyle; how to properly measure blood pressure; what are the treatments for hypertension; what are the indications and side effects of different drugs; how to choose high blood pressure drugs; how to apply hypertension drugs correctly; what symptoms do you need to pay attention to; and other medical content related to hypertension treatment and health care. The third step is the rehabilitation of hypertension mainly for hypertensives who have had complications or dysfunction due to high blood pressure and their relatives and friends. The content includes how to avoid cardiovascular and cerebrovascular complications in hypertensives, how to treat and rehabilitate the hypertensives with complications, how to help the disabled with dysfunction to reenter their jobs or take care of themselves, how to guide relatives and friends to help patients recover together, and other medical content related to the rehabilitation of hypertension.

"Seeing a doctor" is easy to ignore. In a broad sense, it refers to all medical treatment–related content including the process of medical treatment (X-ray examination is required for patients with fractures after plastering in order to confirm the reset situation, which some patients misunderstand as repeated examination), various medical treatment–related systems (the difference between outpatient and emergency), regulations (legal system of body donation), policies (the use of medical insurance), and various medical guidance (how to call an ambulance). Take chest pain as an example. First of all, patients need to know where to go to see a doctor, outpatient or emergency, and the daily routine of the hospital (medical system). If the patient is so unwell and unable to seek medical treatment on his own, then how to call an ambulance? How could he rescue by himself before the arrival of ambulance crews (professional medical guidance)? If the patient arrives at the hospital without medical insurance card in a hurry, how could he seek medical treatment without a medical insurance card? How could he reimburse the medical insurance bureau after the event (medical policy)? During the diagnosis, the doctor judged that the patient needs to complete an electrocardiogram, take a chest radiograph, and do a blood test (medical procedure). The patient was diagnosed with pneumothorax and cured after treatment. The disease may be related to silicosis caused by a large amount of dust in the work environment. To determine whether it is silicosis, the patient should go to the designated institution for identification and clarification according to the Law of the People's Republic of China on the Prevention and Control of Occupational Diseases (medical regulations). On the whole, each part involved in the case is the content of medical communication. Occasionally, the lack of the knowledge mentioned above could be fatal. There was a real case. A patient with a history of coronary heart disease immediately dialed 120 emergency calls during a myocardial infarction and 120 ambulance departed in time. But in the end, because of the neglect of some details, the best rescue time was delayed. It turned out that the patient had just moved to a new community that implemented "human-car diversion" and the address provided by the patient on the phone was the pedestrian entrance, not the entrance to the car. The golden rescue time was delayed for a few minutes to re-find the entrance. Communicating the knowledge of "seeing a doctor" can help people become familiar with the medical treatment process, reduce the waiting time for medical treatment, and help the public master many medical skills.

Finally, talking about "disease cognition" means to spread medical science thoughts and promote the spirit of medical science. It is the highest level and the most overlooked part of medical communication. To prompt the public about the limitations of medicine with a scientific perspective is favorable to establish a good trust of doctors and patients and rational allocation of social medical resources.

Take depression as an example. Some people think it as a flood of beasts and incurable disease, whereas others may think depression is nothing but a disease-free symbol of nothing to look for. These two concepts are wrong. Depression is a very common mental illness that requires attention and care. It requires the necessary psychological and medical treatment as well. If it is not identified and intervened in time, it may have serious consequences. The misunderstanding of this is a popular content for medical communication.

If you have advanced cancers, will you choose to give up any treatment, or go bankrupt and seek medical attention at all costs to continue life? In modern medicine, there is a concept of "survival with cancer," that is, you can think of cancer as a chronic disease as hypertension or diabetes. For those patients who are already in the advanced stage of cancer and have no active treatment, they can coexist with the cancer, taking only symptomatic treatment to soothe the symptoms and reduce the pain of the patient. For those patients at the end of the disease, who are expected to live for less than half a year, they can also carry out hospice care. Physically, try to reduce the patients' pain as much as possible and mentally, help patients and their relatives and friends reduce fear and anxiety and prepare patients to leave. It requires both medical knowledge and humanistic spirit. The famous American doctor, Trudeau said, "*sometimes heal, often help, always comfort.*" Medicine is not omnipotent. Doctors are not omnipotent. Even though today's medicine has reached the molecular level, many diseases are still incurable. The role of medical communication is to help people to treat diseases correctly and rationally, to understand the natural laws of "life and death", to choose the most appropriate treatment and treatment methods, and to apply medical resources reasonably.

3. Relationship between medical communication and health communication

Before the concept of "health communication" was formally introduced, there was an alternative concept in the West, namely "therapeutic communication". Therapeutic communication is closely related to medicine. Until the mid-1970s, health communication, which is a more comprehensive and more abundant concept, has been promoted instead of this restricted one.

Scholars give their own definition of health communication from different angles. Originally proposed by L.D. Jackson in 1992, he believes that "health communication is to use the mass media as a channel to transmit health-related information to prevent disease and promote health. In the process, the mass media is in the medical field. The results have been transformed into public health knowledge prediction and dissemination, and the correct construction of social landscapes to help the audience to establish prevention concepts plays an important role." Then, American scholar E.M. Rogers proposed a definition that "Health communication is a specialty field of communication study that includes the media agenda-setting process for health issues, media advocacy for health, scientific communication among biomedical scientists, doctor–patient communication, and particularly, the design and evaluation of preventive health communication campaigns. The main dependent variables of study in health communication research are usually of unquestioned good: HIV/AIDS prevention, substance abuse prevention and early treatment, improved doctor–patient communication, the effectiveness of media advocacy for health lifestyles, avoidance of unwanted pregnancy, smoking cessation, early detection of cancer, and the prevention of drunk-driving accidents."

He gave a brief explanation of health communication in 1996. "Health communication is any type of human communication whose content is concerned with health" (Rogers, 1996, p. 156). Xu Meiling, a scholar from Taiwan, also discussed the definition of health communication. She considered that "Health communication is the process of people seeking, processing and sharing medical information. It is concerned not only with the process of individuals seeking medical information or the communication between doctors and patients, but also with the flow and processing of information throughout the medical system." The focus of her definition is on the medical field, including the subject, object, and media of health communication. Second, it is multilevel, with individual behavior, as well as systematic behavior.

Health communication is an act of spreading health-related content by four different delivery levels. They are self-individual communication, interpersonal communication, organizational communication, and mass communication. For example, the physical and mental health of individuals is at the level of self-individual, while the relationship between doctor and patient's family is at the interpersonal level, and the relationship between hospital and patient, the on-the-job training of medical staff is at the organizational level and media issue setting. The relationship between media and audience is at the mass level. These four levels do not clearly transmit the subject; they just contain all the health-related content. For this reason, health communication does not emphasize the professionalism of the source of communication to ensure the scientific nature of the content.

From the perspective of scientific communication, medical communication attempts to reduce the unequal information between the two in medical knowledge by building bridges between experts and the public, and to create a scientific culture of society. In this process, it is very clear that the communicator of communication is a professional medical staff. At the same time, it emphasizes the professionalism and scientific nature of the content. Health communication and medical communication are similar in the topic of communication, but there is a fundamental difference. Some examples from the four levels will help us to illustrate the difference between medical communication and health communication.

First, let us see an example at the level of self-individual communication. There was a middle-aged person who was overweight. In order to be healthy, he began to eat only one meal a day. His weight was reduced after two months. He thought this was a very good, effective, and harmless way of losing weight, so he continued. This is the self-individual communication in health communication. For each specific individual, the content of the communication is difficult to control. Those who lack medical common sense will take for granted that some unhelpful and even harmful ways are good for health. Such defects in health communication are difficult to avoid. While in medical communication, if the middle-aged person needs to lose weight, a doctor will complete a health evaluation to confirm whether he is overweight and whether he needs to lose weight at first. Then the doctor will tell him how to scientifically and gradually lose weight, how to lose weight to bring the greatest benefits, and how to avoid the harm of excessive weight loss. It can avoid ambiguity of communication content and the harm to people.

The self-individual communication level in medical communication is the scientific self-propagation under the guidance of professional medical personnel. It can be considered as medical communication if the same person lost his weight guided, approved, and supervised by medical staff.

Second, take an example at the level of interpersonal communication. A diabetic who controlled his blood sugar well by eating only one meal a day and running for two hours a day felt that his blood sugar management experience was very effective. Thus, he shared his experience with his family and other friends with diabetes. This belongs to the human-to-human communication of health, not medical communication. The communicator of medical communication is medical professionals, not patients themselves. The difference is that medical communication should be scientific and draws a universal conclusion, not just a person's own experience and thought. The content of the patient's communication is related to health, so it is in the category of health communication. But in medical communication, this patient is not a professional medical staff and his experience in controlling blood sugar is not accurate and reliable. There are no scientific basis and argument to assert it will play a corresponding role for other patients. So, it clearly does not belong to medical communication. In the field of medical communication, naturally there will also be the possibility of interpersonal communication; as the saying goes, in the process of communication, there is no one to supervise or be responsible for the review of the content of the dissemination. There are too many levels of interpersonal communication, thus there is likely to be a change in the content of the dissemination. It is not possible to guarantee the accuracy and reliability of the dissemination. For example, at the first level of interpersonal communication, the public is informed that the daily amount of salt should be less than 6 g, and to the second level or the third level, or even more, this number may become 16, or become 60, which is very irresponsible. Therefore, there is a phenomenon of human-to-human communication in the field of medical communication, but the interpersonal communication without regulation and organization is not recommended.

Third, take an example at the organizational level. Imagine that a community organized a health lecture, of which the topic was diabetes prevention and health knowledge. If the main speaker is a medical professional, then he can communicate from the mechanism of diabetes, symptoms, harm, and other aspects with vivid elaboration, thus it belongs to the field of medical communication. And if the presenter is only a patient, a teacher, or any other nonprofessional medical personnel, even if the content is the same, the effect is different, because he has not been professionally trained. Then this dissemination can only belong to the field of health communication or organizational communication, not real medical communication, because nonprofessional communicators cannot master the accuracy and knowledge of the content of the communication.

Finally, let's talk about the mass level. At present, a wide variety of media, including new media and self-media, concern about medical and health content. The public generally concern more about themselves and the health of their families than the world political situation. If these media in the dissemination of health content do not have the support of medical professionals, it is best only at the field of health communication or mass communication, not the real sense of medical communication. Medical communication can be in various media, including new media, self-media, but must be carried out and promoted by medical professionals. The content of communication also should be controlled and screened by these medical professionals. The lack of control is easy to cause a variety of miscommunicated content. There are some new media that carry out activities for profit in the name of health; this not only is not beneficial to health, but also has the potential to cause harm to the population, which is one of the reasons why we urgently need to establish the concept of medical communication and the field of medical communication.

In addition to the difference in the subject of communication, the second fundamental difference between medical communication and health communication is the content of the communication. As the communicator of medical communication is medical professionals, the content that is written or identified by medical staff will be scientific and objective. This professional advantage ensures the reliability of the source of medical communication, which is unmatched by traditional health communication scholars. At the same time, medicine has different professions and categories. Therefore, what medical communication scholars spread should be their medical expertise with full professional knowledge, not just general medical knowledge. For instance, a cardiovascular doctor should communicate in the field of cardiovascular medicine, not spread their unfamiliar knowledge in obstetrics and gynecology. Pediatricians should disseminate knowledge in pediatrics. The clinical knowledge and norms of adults are partly different from children, so pediatricians are not suitable for the general dissemination of adult medical knowledge. Therefore, the content of medical communication can be summarized as professional knowledge certified by professionals.

Health communication is a branch of communication, whereas medical communication is a branch of medicine.

4. The characteristics of medical communication

Although in the second section, we discussed the evolution of traditional science communication and explained the three paradigms of traditional science, the fact is that the current scientific communication field in China is still not perfect, so the Deficit Model based on the Public Understanding of Science Paradigm is often the easiest to get policy support and practice. An important reason for this phenomenon is that the science communicators are keen on citizen participation, but the public lack interest in those scientific issues. This shows that we cannot simply put the principles of democratic politics into the field of scientific communication. For example, the energy crisis is a good scientific topic, but the public have limited interest in it. For the public, as long as there is enough gasoline to fuel their cars, they are not as much concerned about the amount of oil left in the world, or whether there is a new energy source to be developed, or what benefits new energy sources can bring to us. Because of the lack of direct relationship, the public will not concern a lot or actively involve themselves.

Unlike general scientific topics, medical and health-related topics are associated with natural public engagement attributes because they are relevant to everyone. From birth to death, people will be inseparable from medical and health-related topics. Starting from how to do prenatal check-ups to how to screen congenital diseases of the fetus, from how to take maternal care to analyze the benefits of taking natural labor and to distinguish which women need a C-section, these prebirth topics are closely related to every couple. And then, there are topics such as follows: how to observe postnatal conditions, how to urge and feed milk, how to decide to feed breast milk or milk powder, how to feed the babies scientifically, how to screen for neonatal diseases, how to bathe newborns, which vaccines are needed and how and where to get them, how to check the nutritional development indicators of children, and how to prevent some common infectious diseases in children. These above-mentioned topics are closely relevant to the puerperal and the newborn. And then in puberty, topics critical to teenagers range from how to guide boys and girls with targeted sexual development counseling to how to smooth through puberty emotional instability, from how to avoid myopia to how to avoid obesity. In adulthood, topics critical to people at the prime of life can be from how to get regular physical examinations to how to develop healthy and beneficial diet and living habits, and how to save oneself when encountering emergencies. When coming to the old age, knowledge from how to screen for common old-age diseases to how to maintain health, from how to exercise properly to how to cultivate good mood, from how to look at death correctly to how to look at the death of a family member, and so on are closely related to the later life of people.

People's whole life is inseparable from medical and health topics, while the public are eager to know all kinds of medical information related to themselves and their families. A person may be apathetic to the latest developments in high-energy physics, but he will always pay attention to the physical and mental health problems of himself and his family. Once a person is sick, he will concern about and consult various medical information including national health insurance–related policies and medical-related regulations and use various communication channels to seek medical information. On July 21, 2015, the Chinese Association of Science and Technology and Baidu held a "Kop China and Baidu" strategic cooperation launch event in Beijing. The two sides jointly released the first "China internet users' popular search behavior report." The report shows that in the first quarter of 2015, searches on popular topics related to health and health care accounted for 57% of all search needs. It can be inferred that medical communication has received widespread attention. Therefore, in the course of the dissemination of medical and health issues, citizens will be more active to participate through various ways and to engage in active dialogue with the medical community, and ultimately a scientific culture conducive to both sides could be created.

The subject of medical communication is medical staff who shoulders the mission of curing sickness and saving patients, which allows them to accurately identify groups that need medical communication and keep track of them. This may be the so-called "precision communication". For those patients who are obese, having high blood pressure or diabetes, medical staff are more likely to prevent the spread and tracking of cardiovascular disease because they are at high risk of cardiovascular disease. For patients with a family history of tumors, medical staff will do more about tumor prevention and screening since their prevalence of tumor is several times higher than in the general population. In the field of medicine, precision medicine is currently promoted. Precision medicine refers to emerging approaches to disease prevention and treatment that take into account an individual's genes, environment, and lifestyle. Similarly, in the field of medical communication, precise medical communication is also required. Precision medical communication is a personalized medical communication that combines an individual's family background, family history, living and eating habits, working environment, and so on. Only precise medical communication can achieve the greatest benefit of the audience. Suppose there are two middle-aged men. They are similar in age, live near to each other, have the same nature of work and similar levels of obesity; meanwhile, both of them usually lack exercise, like desserts and meat, and both like smoking. One has a family history of colorectal cancer, and the other doesn't. When coming to the analysis of the situation from the perspective of medical communication, these two men both have bad habits and diets and lack of exercise, and they are high-risk populations of cardiovascular and cerebrovascular diseases. Because the former has a family history of colorectal cancer, he is also a high-risk group for colorectal cancer. The medical communication for these two men is about the need to have healthy life, diet, and behavior; scientific weight loss methods; and regular screening of cardiovascular disease. The former also needs to be educated to receive regular colorectal cancer screening to have early detection and early treatment, which may not be needed for the latter. This proves that medical communication must be carried out by medical professionals since only professionals can judge the risk factors for different diseases. Then precise medical communication will be provided. The general public does not have such ability.

Medical communication is aimed at people with urgent health needs, such as patients, family members, and sub-healthy people; they are the core of direct contact with medical information. In addition to their own access to useful medical information, they can also radiate it to their loved ones and friends. The information may be disseminated on other issues such as health needs and health systems. Of course, throughout the communication process, professional medical staff are opinion leaders in medical communication and have an important role in leading emotions, spreading issues, and organizing actions. In this form, the transmission and radiation of information belong to the form of interpersonal transmission, but this kind of human-to-human transmission is not a single layer-to-layer transmission. Because a single layer of communication cannot guarantee the accuracy of the content of the communication, loss or even errors are possible in the communication. Interpersonal communication in medical communication does not advocate too many levels of human-to-human communication. Medical communication should be organized and regulated. The person who organizes and supervises is a member of professional medical staff. In the field of medical communication, the subject of communication and the content of transmission are more important than the widespread nature of dissemination. In other words, medical communication pays more attention to the connotation and quality of transmission than to the breadth of transmission. What is needed for medical communication is to pass on medical knowledge to all by medical personnel. The process can be long. To widen the range of spread, more medical personnel are needed to participate or to use more effective means of communication rather than spreading quickly through word-of-mouth in the crowd.

For these reasons, we believe that it is not possible to simply categorize medical communication into the context of scientific communication and fully follow the paradigm of general scientific communication. Medical communication has natural public participation attributes, so we suggest that in practice and theoretical construction, medical communication and general scientific communication should be distinguished.

Chapter 2

Basic Model of Medical Communication

As the communicator of medical communication, the character of medical professionals taking part in the practice of the medical communication is different and inseparable from the usual medical treatment for curing sickness and saving lives. Focusing on the central goal of popularizing medical knowledge, cultivating medical scientific concepts, and shaping social science and culture, the theoretical models of medical communication at different levels have been developed. On the basis of reviewing the model of science communication, we will put forward a contextual participation model under the multi-knowledge framework, which conforms to the current situation of the medical communication practice in China. And then, we will make suggestions on the relationship between the medical communication and research for case analysis.

1. The model of science communication

As mentioned in the first chapter, the practice of science communication has experienced three stages in history: popularization of science, public understanding, and public participation. However, just like the change of social science paradigm, the new paradigm cannot completely replace the old paradigm.[1] So the three paradigms coexist today. At the same time,

---

[1] Kuhn, M. (2004). *The structure of scientific revolution* (J. Wulun & H. Xinhe, Trans.). Beijing: Peking University Press.

due to the complexity and diversity of science communication practice, many kinds of science communication models are applied in different conditions.

1.1. *Types of scientific communication activities*

In October 1999, the British Science Charity Foundation (Wellcome Trust) commissioned a market research company (Research International) to conduct a comprehensive survey of the current status of science communication activities in Britain. The survey analyzed the objectives, audiences, topics, locations, and efficiency of various science communication activities. Based on this analysis, they explored whether these activities needed to be changed, how the public participated in the discussion of science topics and how the communication strategies could be established. This survey had been done through a combination of literature research, quantitative, and qualitative investigation. Qualitative surveys (face-to-face interviews and telephone interviews) and quantitative surveys (telephone interviews and online surveys) are mainly concerned with the themes, objectives, role of organizers, efficiency, evaluation criteria and funding sources of past scientific communication activities, strategies for future scientific communication activities, experiences of other scientific communication activities, and views on science communication activities. After the investigation, various types of scientific communication activities were summarized in the report "Science and the Public: Atlas of Scientific Communication Activities". Of the survey, the target audience including the general public and policy makers, the communication objectives including promoting public interest, deepening scientific understanding and influencing scientific policy, and the types of scientific communication activities all showed their diversity and complexity (Figure 2.1).

At the same time, the use of media is also rich and diverse in different scientific fields. There are traces of scientific communication in the domains of mass media (such as television, magazines), new media (network, mobile media), scientific competitions, and public lectures. Finally, the report argues that hands-on and interactive approaches are efficient for science communication. Interactive science communication activities can break the barriers between the public and the scientific

**Overall picture:
activities**

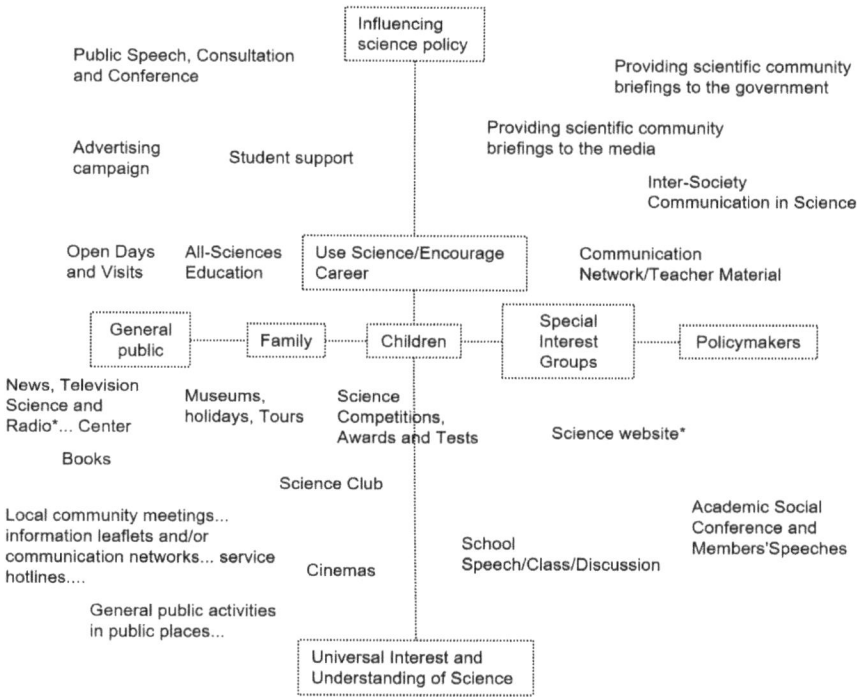

Public Speech, Consultation
and Conference

Influencing
science policy

Providing scientific community
briefings to the government

Advertising
campaign

Student support

Providing scientific community
briefings to the media

Inter-Society
Communication in Science

Open Days
and Visits

All-Sciences
Education

Use Science/Encourage
Career

Communication
Network/Teacher Material

General
public

Family

Children

Special
Interest
Groups

Policymakers

News, Television
Science and
Radio*... Center

Museums,
holidays, Tours

Science
Competitions,
Awards and Tests

Science website*

Books

Science Club

Local community meetings...
information leaflets and/or
communication networks... service
hotlines....

Cinemas

School
Speech/Class/Discussion

Academic Social
Conference and
Members'Speeches

General public activities
in public places...

Universal Interest and
Understanding of Science

* The readership is broader than shown.

Figure 2.1   Atlas of types of scientific communication activities.

Source of data: Science and the Public: Mapping Science Communication Activities. Prepared by
Research International.[2]

community and establish their dialogue mechanism. However, this
interaction should be tailored to local conditions at the right times. The
scientific community should and has begun to understand the public,
rather than just asking the public to "work harder" alone. Some of the
public has not been covered, so more efforts are needed in this regard.
Media using has both opportunities and challenges in science

---

[2] https://www.gov.uk/government/uploads/system/uploads/attachment_data/file/260650/
science-and-public-mapping-science-communication-activities.pdf

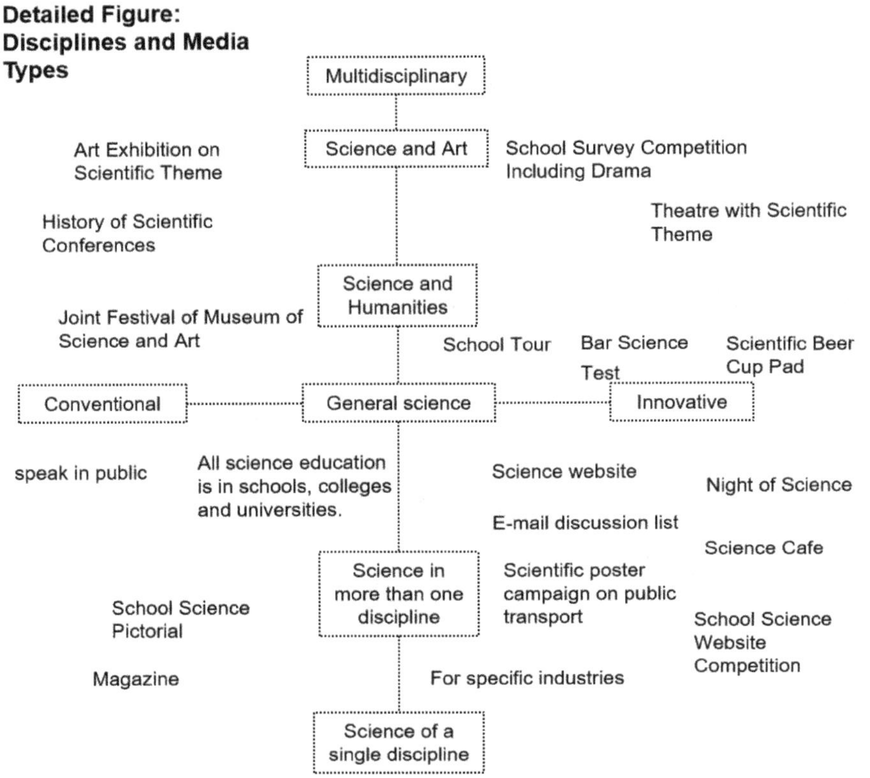

Detailed Figure:
Disciplines and Media
Types

Figure 2.2   Discipline and media use in science communication activities.

Source of data: Science and the public: Mapping science communication activities. Prepared by Research International.[3]

communication, so improving the relationship between scientific community and media is conducive to the development of science communication (Figure 2.2).[3]

The complexity and diversity of science communication activities also exist in the practice of science communication in China. The results of the Chinese Citizens' Scientific Literacy Survey conducted by the Chinese Association of Science and Technology over the years showed

---

[3] https://www.gov.uk/government/uploads/system/uploads/attachment_data/file/260650/science-and-public-mapping-science-communication-activities.pdf

that the public's access to scientific information is diversified, and the levels of the infrastructure and the science activities of science populariza-tion were also improving steadily. From March to August in 2015, the Chinese Association of Science and Technology launched the ninth sampling survey on the scientific literacy of Chinese citizens, covering 31 provinces, autonomous regions and municipalities directly under the Central Government in the mainland of China. According to the survey published in September 2015 (Table 2.1), the proportion of citizens using the Internet and mobile Internet to obtain scientific and technological information reached 53.4%, which ranked more than twice of 26.6% in 2010, surpassing newspapers (38.5%) and second only to televisions (93.4%). Internet and mobile internet had become the first channel for citizens with scientific quality to obtain scientific and technological infor-mation, through which up to 91.2% of them obtained the information. As a traditional mass media, television is still the main channel for citizens to obtain scientific and technological information. The percentage of citizens using TV to obtain scientific and technological information was 93.4%, which was slightly higher than that in 2010 (87.5%), far less than the growth rate of the proportion of citizens accessing the information through the Internet. In terms of popular science facilities, the opportunities had increased in access to scientific knowledge and scientific and technologi-cal information through popular science facilities for citizens; also, the utilization rate of popular science facilities had been improved. In the past year, the proportions of citizens visiting all kinds of popular science ven-ues are: science and technology museums (22.7%) and nature museums (22.1%). The proportions of visiting popular science places nearby are: book reading room (34.3%), popular science gallery, or propaganda board (20.7%). Comparing with the data of visiting rate of non-formal science education places in American Science and Engineering Index (2014), the utilization of popular science facilities in China is similar to that in the United States (25% of American citizens visited science and technology museums and other science and technology venues, 28% of them visited nature museums in 2012).

However, it was not clear whether the effectiveness of these scientific communication practices could be regarded as "success". One of the important reasons was that there was no consensus on the goal of science

Table 2.1   The use of public science popularization channels in China in 2005, 2010, and 2015.

Survey items		Multiple choice (%)			
Channel utilization	**Channel**	**2005**	**2007**	**2010**	**Illustration**
Investigation on Citizens' Access to Scientific and Technological Information in China	Television	91.0	90.2	87.5	The figures in the table show the proportion of public access to scientific and technological information through these channels.
	Newspaper	44.9	60.2	50.1	
	Interpersonal communication	48.7	34.7	43.0	
	Internet	7.9	10.7	26.6	
	Radio broadcast	22.4	20.6	24.6	
	General magazine	Merge into news-papers	9.7	12.2	
	Books	10.2	11.9	11.9	
	Scientific journals	9.5	13.2	10.5	
	Other channels	7.9	/	/	
Investigation on Citizens' Visits to Popular Science Infrastructure in China	Zoo, aquarium, botanical garden	30.3	51.9	57.9	The figures in the table show the proportion of visitors to such popular science infrastructure in the past year.
	Book reading room	29.2	43.7	54.5	
	public library	26.7	41.0	50.3	
	Popular science gallery, publicity column	36.7	46.8	48.7	
	Science and technology demonstration site, popular science activity station	30.9	29.1	35.5	
	Industrial and agricultural production park	/	30.0	34.2	
	Science and technology museum and other venues like this	9.3	16.7	27.0	
	Museum of natural history	7.1	13.9	21.9	
	Art galleries, exhibition galleries	11.2	17.5	26.4	
	Laboratories of universities and scientific research institutions	/	2.7	11.2	

Table 2.1   (*Continued*)

Survey items		Multiple choice (%)			
Channel utilization	Channel	2005	2007	2010	Illustration
Public Participation in Popular Science Activities in China	Science Week, Science Popularization Day	11.9	14.7	23.8	The figures in the table show the proportion of the public who participated in such popular science activities in the past year.
	Science and technology training	30.8	35.2	35.6	
	Science and technology consultation	30.4	32.4	31.4	
	Popular science lecture	23.9	25.8	29.4	
	Science and technology exhibition	/	21.3	25.1	
	Popular science publicity and broadcasting activities	11.6	13.8	13.7	

communication. Therefore, Bruce Lewenstein, Professor of Science Communication at Cornell University, wrote the four common models of scientific communication.[4]

1.2. *Four different models*

1.2.1. *Model 1: The deficit model*

The deficit model was proposed by John Durant, a Professor of Public Understanding of Science at Imperial College of Science, Technology and Medicine. He was also the Editor-in-Chief of *Public Understanding of Science* and the first professor of public understanding of science appointed by Royal Society of England. Durant thought that the public was short of scientific literacy and interest in science, so it was necessary to popularize and educate scientific knowledge to the public. In short, the main characteristic of deficit models was the public education by scientists. For example, since the 1970s, the National Science Council of the United States had

---

[4]Lewenstein, B. (2003). *Models of public communication of science and technology.* Retrieved from https://edisciplinas.usp.br/pluginfile.php/43775/mod_resource/content/1/ Texto/Lewenstein%202003.pdf

regularly measured the level of scientific knowledge of the public. The Committee was disappointed to find that only 10% of Americans could define a "molecule", while more than half believed that humans and dinosaurs were present on Earth at the same time. Based on these findings, the Committee concluded that only 5% of American citizens were scientifically literate and only 20% were interested in science, while others were referred to as "the rest of the population". The deficit model confirms that when the public's scientific literacy improves, it will support the development and application of science and technology in the country. Therefore, the early deficit model had a strong government-oriented color.

However, critics of the deficit model believed that this model presupposes some ideas: scientific knowledge was absolutely reliable, playing a supreme role in modern life; scientific knowledge could only flow from top to bottom; the improvement of scientific knowledge level was the only way to solve the problem of public alienating, doubting or even rejecting science, and so on.[5] More scholars pointed out that the deficit model did not take context into account. Learning theory shows that only when facts and theories were meaningful in life could people grasp them best. For example, residents in water-polluted areas could quickly grasp complex terminology related to water pollution. Some scholars pointed out that the fatal weakness of the deficit model was that it tried to impose the cognitive model of occupational science onto the public's understanding of science. Durant himself also realized that the deficit model accused the public of not taking their place in the relationship between science and society, and it also did not realize that the inconsistency between experts and the public in understanding might be due to the redefinition or reestablishment of science in specific contexts. It produced a one-way propagation process between science and the public, which is of no value or even of destruction, so, the public is skeptical about science in the process.

We assumed that the deficit model was applied to medical communication, then it was top-down propaganda of medical knowledge. Just as the deficit model in scientific communication characterized by scientists educating the public, the deficit model in medical communication was

---

[5] Fujun, R., & Jiequan, Z. (2012). *Science and technology dissemination and popularization course*. Beijing: China Science and Technology Press.

characterized by professional medical personnel educating the public. However, if only through education, it was very questionable whether the public was interested and how much they can be accepted. Figuratively speaking, the deficit model was similar to spoon-feeding education in primary and secondary school. I forced the transfer or education of medical knowledge to you in a variety of ways, regardless of whether this method was effective or whether the content was appropriate. Not to mention how effective it was for the public to acquire medical knowledge in this mode. Under the cramming education, even if the public acquired some medical knowledge, he might not understand the knowledge he had acquired very well. Such education is deficient congenitally. Let us take iodine supplementation for example. Iodine is one of the essential trace elements in human body. If iodine deficiency occurs, it may cause abortion, stillbirth, congenital malformation, neuromotor dysfunction in the fetus, hypothyroidism and goiter in the newborn, goiter in the childhood, hypothyroidism, subclinical cretinism, mental retardation and physical development disorder in adolescence, and goiter and its complications, hypothyroidism, and mental retardation in adulthood. If iodine is excessive, it may cause hyperthyroidism and other problems. In China, there are many iodine deficiency areas where iodine needs to be supplemented. Many authoritative media often propagated that the residents of our country should use iodized salt. In the Reform Plan of Salt Industry System, it was also stipulated that the coverage rate of qualified iodized salt should be over 90%. That is the deficit model in medical communication if we do not consider the regional issues of whether all regions are iodine deficiency areas, and the reason why iodine supplement should be used to publicize the whole population, and advertise for those to supply iodine, but not to tell them how to supply iodine scientifically and what harm iodine deficiency has and does to people. On the one hand, the public was told to supply iodine. But it was not clear how many people cared about the importance of iodine to the human body. Many of the public might think that iodine deficiency had nothing to do with themselves, so they did not care about it. On the other hand, some of the public may take iodine actively as required, but some of them might not be suitable for iodine supplementation. Excessive iodine supplementation may also lead to other diseases; thus this kind of medical communication is undoubtedly useless and may even be harmful.

Applying the deficit model to medical communication, as it has presupposed its supremacy, it shows its absolute authority when it spreads and propagates, but ignores whether the public is concerned about it and how much knowledge can be accepted. Therefore, even if the content of dissemination is very reliable, the effect of dissemination is also debatable. For example, hypertension is a very common chronic disease. According to the 12th Five-Year Plan sample survey of hypertension published by the State Health Planning Commission in 2017, the prevalence of hypertension among adults in China was 23%, and the number of adults was 243 million, which meant that one in four adults suffered from hypertension. The awareness rate, treatment rate, control rate, and treatment control rate of hypertension were 42.7%, 38.3%, 14.5%, and 38.0% respectively. The awareness rate, treatment rate, and control rate of hypertension in rural areas were lower than those in urban areas. From this survey, we can see that the prevalence of hypertension in Chinese population is high and the awareness rate is low. It is very urgent and necessary to improve people's awareness of hypertension. In order to improve the prevalence rate of hypertension knowledge, local students in the school were popularized the knowledge of hypertension through books. Let's see how it works. First of all, primary school students are generally not concerned about the common diseases of adults such as hypertension because they are not high-risk groups of hypertension and have low incidence of hypertension. Secondly, pupils' cognition and cognitive ability are still at a developmental stage, and they cannot reach the adult's cognitive level. Because of their limited understanding ability, the degree of understanding will not be very high. And If only books are used to popularize medical knowledge, the effect will not be very good. If the communication was carried out in the form of image cartoons or interactive lectures, the effect might be increased significantly.

Based on the defects of the deficit model, the following three models have been proposed successively.

1.2.2. *Model 2: The contextual model*

The basic view of contextual model is that the public is not an empty bottle waiting for knowledge to be injected; instead, the absorption and processing of information will be influenced by social environment and personal psychology. Therefore, previous experience, cultural context and personal environment will influence the public's view of science. In the process of science communication, we are not facing a single audience, but a pluralistic audience with different cultural backgrounds. Why do they need scientific information? Under what circumstances do they need scientific information? Therefore, we need a model of disseminating scientific information to different audiences at different times and in different ways, according to different contexts. This is the contextual model. The contextual model is widely used in the fields of audience perception, such as health communication, risk communication, and risk perception.

First of all, the contextual model takes into account many factors of personal and environment, including life stage, personality, and interpersonal relationship, which will affect the reception of information. Secondly, the social system and media presentation will also deepen or weaken the public's attention to certain issues. Therefore, contextual model scholars use modern market segmentation method to analyze the scientific literacy of different groups and disseminate different scientific knowledge.

We give some appropriate examples to illustrate how the contextual model apply to medical communication in the following.

For example, Tibet is a famous tourist destination, while Potala Palace is a place where many people need pilgrimage. But Tibet is a typical plateau area. Compared with the plain area, the oxygen content there is obviously low. Many people are likely to have altitude sickness because of lack of oxygen for the first time. High-altitude reaction is a common disease in plateau area, including common symptoms of headache, insomnia, loss of appetite, fatigue, dyspnea, etc. Generally speaking, 50%–75% of the people in the plain experienced altitude reaction when they entered the plateau above 3000 m suddenly, but the symptoms gradually disappeared after 3–10 days of acclimation. Acute high-altitude reaction is very likely to result in high-altitude pulmonary edema and/or high-altitude brain edema. If we do not pay attention to it, we may lose our lives. Because of the particularity of plateau reaction, many people going to travel will be very concerned about how to prevent altitude sickness, and they will pay attention to the medical knowledge of it. Considering the focus of these groups, the contextual model of medical communication is to popularize medical knowledge among those who are going to travel to the plateau about how to prevent from and treat with the plateau reaction after the plateau reaction occurs. Compared with the deficit model, at least it focuses on the needs of the public, and its publicity and popularization shoot the arrow at the target.

For another example, chronic hepatitis B, or hepatitis B for short, is caused by infection with hepatitis B virus. China is a high incidence area of hepatitis B. According to statistics, the number of hepatitis B virus carriers in China is as high as 120 million, and the number of cases is more than 30 million. A considerable number of hepatitis B patients present family clustering characteristics. The incidence of cirrhosis and hepatocellular carcinoma in patients with hepatitis B was significantly higher than that in non-hepatitis B patients. Hepatitis B virus listed as a carcinogen of Class I in October 2017. Therefore, for a large number of hepatitis B virus carriers, patients, or the members of their families, they are quite concerned about the health knowledge of hepatitis B. They want to know which way hepatitis B is transmitted, how to avoid infection or the common complications of hepatitis B, and how to keep healthy after getting hepatitis B. Then combining with their concerns, they, on the one hand, communicate the importance of hepatitis B vaccine injection in the population, on the other hand, publicize the importance of regular physical examination and liver protection for the people who are already carriers of hepatitis B. That is a good combination of public needs, and also a reflection of the contextual model.

Sometimes, we will find that the concern about the topic will change with the influence of personal environment or personal psychology. That is to say, the context may change. For example, recently someone's friend, a middle-aged man, whose age and work are similar to him, developed lung cancer suddenly. During this period of time, he will be very concerned about various medical knowledge about lung cancer. After a while, another friend of his died of acute myocardial infarction, then he turned to the medical knowledge of myocardial infarction instead of the lung cancer that he had paid attention to previously. Therefore, the context will change with the environment and psychology around the individual. However, in the contextual model, we also need to consider whether the individual needs to focus on. The context problem is whether it is the real medical issue that needs to be concerned about. For example, if the middle-aged man mentioned above usually does not smoke or drink, is of moderate size, not overweight or obese, has no history of chronic diseases, such as hypertension, diabetes, hyperlipidemia, and has no history of lung cancer or cardiovascular and cerebrovascular diseases in his family, then he is not at high risk for cardiovascular diseases such as lung cancer or myocardial infarction. However, his family has a history of colorectal cancer, and he himself has a long history of constipation, so he is of a high-risk group of colorectal cancer. He should know or master the relevant medical knowledge of colorectal cancer rather than the knowledge of lung cancer and cardiovascular and cerebrovascular diseases.

In addition, many critics pointed out that the contextual model was only an upgraded version of the deficit model, both of which equated "public understanding of science" with "public appreciation of the benefits of science to society". Since the 1980s, science communication scholars have begun to emphasize layman knowledge and public participation, thus putting forward the following two models.

1.2.3. *Model 3: The lay expertise model*

The contextual model recognized the value of scientific knowledge, but did not deny the complexity of scientific knowledge dissemination, and the lay expertise model recognized the importance of lay knowledge or local knowledge in solving scientific and technological problems. This model is also called as "the local knowledge model" or "the reflexivity model". The lay expertise model emphasized that the dissemination of scientific knowledge should be based on the existing layman knowledge structure in the community, recognizing the value of local knowledge owned by the public, rather than simply assuming that the public should accept scientific knowledge without doubt, which resulted in the loss of public trust in science. The lay expertise model was a controversial scientific knowledge dissemination model. First of all, we need to admit that in addition to the knowledge created by scientists in the laboratory through formal scientific research, in some developing countries with long history, they have accumulated considerable practical experience in long-term production and life practices, and gradually matured and transformed them into relevant knowledge after years of accumulation. It was not formed by the traditional scientific methods recognized by scientists today, but it was proved to be effective in practice. It is one of the important ways to improve the public's scientific literacy to certify and theorize these layman's or informal skills and knowledge through scientific methods so that they can enter the field of formal education and communication.

This model was very popular in the culture with local knowledge system. For example, traditional calendars in China (Lunar calendar), traditional Chinese medicine (TCM, Chinese medicine), and Tibetan traditional medicine (Tibetan medicine) were regarded as representatives of local knowledge. These folk knowledge with non-standardized features were derived from long-term production and living practice. They were controversial but effective in many cases, so it had been inherited and played an important role in people's daily life. The lay expertise model considers exactly how to incorporate the influence of indigenous knowledge into the process of scientific communication. In fact, more and more countries have realized the importance of disseminating the indigenous knowledge of the mainstream society through the formal education system. For example, the National Science and Technology Development Bureau of Thailand started in 2002 to study how to use modern science to explain the formation process and methods of local foods, herbs, and handicrafts. The research results were submitted to the government to formulate corresponding policies to promote the social and economic development.

Let's see what it looks like if only a lay expertise model is applied to medical communication. In the previous paragraph, we mentioned that TCM was the representative of local knowledge in China. Traditional Chinese medicine came into being in primitive society. During the Spring and Autumn Period and the Warring States Period, the theory of traditional Chinese medicine was formed basically, and then it was summarized and developed in successive dynasties. Traditional Chinese medicine carries the experience and theoretical knowledge of ancient Chinese people's struggle against diseases. It is a medical theoretical system gradually formed and developed through long-term medical practice under the guidance of ancient simple materialism and spontaneous dialectics. Based on Yin Yang and five elements, Chinese medicine regards the human body as a unity of Qi, form, and spirit. It explores the etiology, disease, location, analysis of pathogenesis, changes in the organs, meridians, joints, Qi, blood, and body fluid, and it judges the positive and negative growth and decline of the disease through the method of "look, listen, question and feel the pulse", which are the four points of diagnosis and consultation. If we incorporate the knowledge influence of TCM into the process of medical communication, it is the lay expertise model in medical communication. It should be said that traditional Chinese medicine is the quintessence of traditional medicine, and there are many successful cases and experiences that can be learned and carried forward. However, how to disseminate and whether all the knowledge of traditional Chinese medicine is suitable for medical communication is also worth exploring. For example, TCM advocates the two concepts of the same treatment for different diseases and the same treatment for different diseases. Same treatment for different diseases refers to the principle that different diseases have the same pathogenesis in the course of their development, so they are treated by the same method. Different diseases can be treated in the same way, depending neither on the etiology nor on the syndrome. The key lies in identifying whether different diseases have the same pathogenesis. Only when the pathogenesis is the same, can the same treatment be adopted. Different treatment of the same disease refers to the fact that the treatments of the same disease will be different because of different stages, pathogenesis, symptoms, seasons of onset, and physique of individuals during the process of the disease. These two concepts have been handed down from generation to generation in Chinese traditional medicine for thousands of years and are highly respected by the Chinese medical profession. But a large part of traditional Chinese medicine pays attention to experience, which is not well understood and mastered by the general population. If we vigorously publicize different treatment for same diseases and the same treatment for different diseases among the general public, many people may not understand, or misunderstand them. Taking cold for instance, traditional Chinese medicine classifies it into wind-cold type and wind-heat type. Wind-cold cold is caused by the external attack of wind-cold evil and the loss of lung-qi; wind-heat cold is caused by the evil offence of wind-heat and the lung-qi failing to keep on good terms. Wind-cold and wind-heat medicines are completely different, but ordinary people cannot distinguish between wind-cold and wind-heat. They have the idea of treating different diseases with the same treatment, so they think they can use the same drug to deal with them. But they do not know that the same drug may have completely different effects on two types of cold. The wrong drug may also aggravate the symptoms and the course of cold. Therefore, the accuracy and comprehensibility of the content should also be taken into account when applying the lay expertise model to medical communication.

Although the local knowledge model emphasizes the public's possession of layman's knowledge and demonstrates the equal relationship between the public and scientists to a certain extent, which has been supported by many scholars, it has also been criticized by many scholars. This model gives priority to local knowledge over modern scientific knowledge, so it is considered as "anti-science". At the same time, it distinguishes scientific knowledge from layman knowledge, which in fact may exacerbate the tension between the public and scientists.

1.2.4. *Model 4: The public participation model (the public engagement model)*

The public participation model requires that the public participate in the discussion of scientific and technological issues in a democratic system to ensure the democratization and openness of public policy decision-making, at the same time, to improve the public's scientific literacy in the process of participating in the discussion, and to ensure the public's understanding of science, technology, and research. In the process of participation, the public will be aware of the relationship between science and society. This model emphasizes that the public should take the initiative to participate in the setting up of the scientific agenda, and engage in dialogue with the scientific community, so as to establish a democratic mechanism for public participation in scientific decision-making. So this model is also called the democratic model or the dialogue model. Durant, who proposed the deficit model, also saw the limitations of the deficit model in his later period. He believed that the missing model and the democratic model could coexist as two models of public understanding of science.

Since the second half of the 20th century, the development of science and technology has not only improved human life, but also brought anxiety and fear to the public. The development and application of nuclear energy, genetically modified food, cloning technology, and many other frontier technologies have caused widespread social controversy. Health and safety risks and ethical challenges associated with these technologies have created a crisis of public trust in science. Therefore, the government and scientists are gradually aware of the importance of developing scientific dialogue. The public participation model, which emphasizes the two-way dialogue between experts and non-experts, is widely considered to be superior to the deficit model. In brief, the deficit model is more likely to be suitable in some areas, such as formal science education, while the democratic model or public participation model is more suitable in other areas, such as public debate on environmental issues relative to genetically modified foods.

Shall we imagine applying the public participation model to medical communication? For example, a patient was found to have early gastric cancer and needed treatment. Doctors talk with patients and their families, communicating and informing them that there are several treatment options available, the advantages of each treatment, which complications are likely to occur, the current situation of patients, and which treatment is more appropriate. In the process of communicating and discussing with family members, the two sides finally reached an agreement to choose the most suitable treatment for patients. This is the model of public participation in medical communication. Facing the same patient, if the doctor simply tells the patient and his family that they must choose a treatment method without any communication and discussion, then that is the deficit model in medical communication. In this scenario, we can see that the model of public participation in medical communication may be more easily understood and adopted by the public. However, in the public participation model, it is also necessary to take into account the degree of public participation, the basic cultural level of the public and the acceptability of knowledge. Imagine that in the process of communicating with the patient's family members, if the family members do not participate at all, it is not a real public participation model, but more like the deficit model. Or the public participation models will do harm to the patients when their family members, based on their own one-sided knowledge, ask doctors to choose a treatment that is totally inappropriate or impossible? For example, a patient with advanced cancer, whose general condition was very poor and life was dying, was advised to his family members to take palliative treatment. However, in the public participation model, in the process of communication between doctors and the patients' families, the family members asked the doctor for the only way of surgical treatment to the patient, regardless of the patient's current basic situation, then was the final treatment mean in the hands of doctors or family members? Which is the decisive factor in the following? Who is more powerful, can be persuaded by the other, or who is more scientific, more rational, or more based? Is it necessary to adopt the opinions of family members (the public) in the public participation model? These are the problems we need to think about when we apply the public participation model in medical communication.

It should be said that the model of public participation conforms to the requirements of social democratization and promotes the change of scientific communication concept, but it also faces many doubts. For example, the public participation model is more like a political science model of science and public relations than a science communication model. At the same time, this model is also regarded as having the tendency of "anti-science". These are the questions that the public participation model needs to answer.

2. Medical communication model

As mentioned in the first chapter, although there is a certain subordination between medical communication and scientific communication, due to the natural public participation attribute of medical communication, the scientific communication model introduced in the first section cannot fully and effectively guide the practice of medical communication. First of all, because health issues are closely related to everyone, the public does not completely or absolutely lack medical knowledge. Everyone has some health experience and common sense more or less. Secondly, the emergence of disease and the maintenance of health have a strong context of personal life, which needs to consider individual life experience, social environment, and cultural impact. For example, the health demands of residents in Hengduan Mountain Area of Yunnan may differ greatly from those of residents in Shanghai. Thirdly, considering the influence of traditional Chinese medical culture, the "layman knowledge" (such as health preserving knowledge of traditional Chinese Medicine) of modern medical knowledge is widely spread. Therefore, the public has local medical knowledge in varying degrees, which is also a problem to be considered when conducting medical communication. Finally, the ultimate goal of medical communication is to improve the health level of the whole society. Therefore, the public should take part in the decision-making of medical science. Therefore, none of the above four models can cover all aspects of medical communication practice. Based on a comprehensive review of the current practice of medical communication in China, we propose the multi-expertise contextual engagement model.

First of all, we need to fully consider the multiple medical health knowledge system of Chinese residents. In the past thousands of years of Chinese civilization, traditional Chinese medicine, Tibetan medicine, and other local traditional medical system knowledge have been deeply rooted in people's minds through oral communication, community communication, book communication, and other ways. While these traditional medical systems have solved some problems, there are also many disputes. Let's give some typical examples. As everyone knows, after giving birth to a child, the mother has to rest for a month. Confinement can be traced back to the book of rites of the Western Han Dynasty, known as "within the month", which is a necessary ritual behavior after childbirth. Confinement is the process of helping the parturient to recuperate and adapt to the role of the new mother as soon as possible, and it is also the key period of helping the parturient to pass through the physiological and psychological transition of life smoothly. So what should the parturient do during her confinement? There are many classic practices handed down from the older generation, and there is no scientific basis for the correctness of these practices. For example, the older generation said that during the confinement period, you must "cover up", not catch cold, not be exposed to the wind, not be able to take a bath, not to wash your hair, of course, not to turn on the air conditioner, even in the hot summer. In the past few years, a tragedy happened in a certain place, that is, the mother listened to the idea that she must "cover up" during the period of confinement. During the ultra-high temperature in July, the mother also wrapped up very tightly, dressed in thick clothes, covered with thick quilts, and did not open air conditioning, windows, without showers, which eventually led to heat stroke of the mother, finally being announced no cure after being sent to the hospital. For another example, many people think that traditional Chinese medicine is safer than western medicine and has no side effects. It's not clear why people had this idea and where this idea came from. It may have been passed down from generation to generation. As a result, many people like to eat traditional Chinese medicine after getting sick, and for health preservation. We don't mean to belittle traditional Chinese medicine here, but all drugs have certain side effects and are not absolutely safe. The "kidney disease of Chinese herbal medicine" which caused great furor in the past few years is a typical example. "Kidney disease of Chinese herbal medicine" in that year was caused by aristolochic acid contained in some Chinese herbal ingredients. There are a lot of traditional Chinese medicines containing aristolochic acid, including more than a dozen kinds, such as Guanmutong, Guangfangji, Qingmuxiang, Zhushalian, Tianxianteng, Asarum, Fangji, Huaitong, and Dujuan. So the Hong Kong Department of health has banned the sale of traditional Chinese medicine containing aristolochic acid in 2004. In 2005, the national pharmacopoeia of China banned three kinds of Chinese medicine with high content of aristolochic acid, i.e. Guanmutong, Guangfangji, and Qingmuxiang. In the list of carcinogens published by the World Health Organization in 2017, aristolochic acid and plants containing it are included in a class of carcinogens. It can be seen that traditional Chinese medicine is not absolutely safe, and it needs to be used under the guidance and supervision of doctors. In these cases, we can see that the public has a lot of medical knowledge from the traditional system, from the ancestral ideas of grandparents, fathers, and mothers, and there is no solid scientific and medical basis, which is very questionable in practical application. In recent years, there is another phenomenon worthy of attention. With the development of network and information technology, people may search for medical knowledge through the Internet. For example, a middle-aged man recently suffered from poor appetite, weight loss, and general weakness. He didn't have time to go to the hospital for examination, and there were no doctors or friends to consult. Online search is the easiest. So, he went online and searched through search engines. Once he found out that gastric cancer had these symptoms, he took it for granted that he had gastric cancer. But there are many other diseases that may have these symptoms. As for the cause of the disease, it can only be determined through regular medical tests. It doesn't confirm to be gastric cancer. For another example, diabetes is a group of metabolic diseases characterized by hyperglycemia. Seven large-scale epidemiological surveys on diabetes conducted in China showed that the prevalence of diabetes was gradually increasing. In the latest, the 7th epidemiological survey conducted in 2013, the prevalence of type 2 diabetes in the population over 18 years old in China reached 10.4%, among which men were higher than women. That means one in 10 adults was diabetic. Therefore, it is necessary to popularize the medical knowledge about diabetes. And the medical knowledge about diabetes on the Internet is also overwhelming and accessible. One patient with diabetes took oral hypoglycemic drugs but the effect was not good. The doctor required him to inject a certain amount of insulin every day. The patients' blood sugar was well controlled since insulin was used instead. But this patient always felt that it was a little trouble to use insulin every day. So, one day, this patient found some kind of health care product to reduce blood sugar by checking on the Internet. The health care product was boasted how effective its hypoglycemic effect was, and the patient himself felt that it was troublesome to use insulin, so he stopped using insulin without permission and changed it into the health care product recommended on the Internet, which eventually caused blood sugar surge and coma and the patient was sent to the hospital for emergency treatment. Fortunately, the rescue was successful and a life was recovered. These cases are all based on the harm of medical knowledge obtained from Internet search. It is the bounden duty of medical communicators to correct the wrong views of health through the dissemination of scientific medical knowledge. However, there was no denying that many of these "local knowledge" and "layman knowledge" still played a positive role. Therefore, the so-called "grandma doctor" (that is, the elder's health care knowledge), "Internet doctor" (that is, the medical health knowledge based on the Internet) and other phenomena were very common. Because most of the people do not have the attribute of medical knowledge, the medical staff who carry out medical communication first need to ensure that the content of the communication must be accurate. At the same time, we need to consider how to spread the modern medical science knowledge while fully taking into account the existing multiple knowledge structure of the object of communication. We should try to avoid the conflict between multiple knowledge and realize the truly effective medical communication.

Secondly, we need to give full consideration to the context of our residents' health issues. China is the third largest country in the world, with a vast area and different cultural customs and living habits. The health problem is deeply rooted in the local culture, so it is necessary for medical communicators to take full pre-research, to understand the local folk culture and health demands, and spread medical knowledge according to different people and different places. For example, cardiovascular disease is a common disease of middle-aged and old people, with the characteristics of high incidence, high disability rate, high mortality, low control rate, low standard rate, so called three high and two low. According to *China cardiovascular disease report 2017*, the mortality rate of cardiovascular disease in China ranked first in 2017, higher than that of tumor and other diseases. The proportion of deaths has reached about 45%. That is to say, in China, two out of every five deaths are from cardiovascular diseases. And the number of cardiovascular patients is as high as 290 million. The morbidity and mortality of cardiovascular diseases are still on the rise. It should be said that cardiovascular disease is a kind of disease that needs to be paid much attention, and also a kind of disease that needs to carry out medical dissemination and medical science popularization. The main risk factors of cardiovascular disease include overweight, obesity, lack of exercise, high salt, high oil diet, etc. It is very necessary and popular to carry out the prevention and control of cardiovascular diseases in the target population, such as in major cities. It is a kind of medical communication which is very suitable for the needs of the public. Once upon a time, there were medical science popularization workers who went deep into the mountainous areas of Yunnan Province to popularize the prevention and treatment of cardiovascular diseases for rural residents. Due to the lack of investigation on the diet, life, and behavior of local residents in advance, when they had arrived the area, it was found that the diet structure of local residents was low in crude food and oil. In addition, they often need to climb mountains at ordinary times, thus the amount of daily exercise and the number of days of exercise per week were sufficient, and cardiovascular problems were not common. Therefore, they failed to take proper medicine and effectively communicate. For another example, Keshan disease is a kind of local cardiomyopathy. It was first discovered in Keshan city of Heilongjiang Province in 1935. The main cause is the lack of selenium in the diet. It was reported that at least 700 million people in China live in selenium deficient areas. The spread of prevention and control knowledge of Keshan disease will not only be popular, but also benefit the local residents. But if we go to non-selenium deficient areas or even selenium rich areas, such as Enshi in Hubei Province, Rugao in Jiangsu Province and other areas to carry out the prevention and control science popularization of Keshan disease, it is just for the purpose of science popularization, which is not suitable. In addition, when conducting medical communication, we also need to consider the needs of different genders and different age groups. Taking gender as an example, people of different genders have different physiological structures. For example, prostate is a unique organ for men, while uterus and ovary are unique organs for women. If we carry out science popularization of "ovarian cancer" in men and "prostate cancer" in women, even if it is not a joke, the benefit it can bring is little. At the same time, people of different genders and body structures have different concerns and health demands. For example, lectures on "breast disease" and "uterine disease" and lectures on prevention of "prostatic hyperplasia" are given to adult women and men, respectively, which is a good topic to be selected, meeting the context and needs of health issues of different gender groups. People of different genders have different disease spectrum. Taking the incidence of cancer in men and women as an example, the top ten tumors in men in China are lung cancer, stomach cancer, liver cancer, esophageal cancer, colorectal cancer, bladder cancer, prostate cancer, lymphoma, brain nervous system tumor, and pancreatic cancer, while the top ten tumors in women are breast cancer, lung cancer, colorectal cancer, stomach cancer, thyroid cancer, cervical cancer, liver cancer, esophageal cancer, uterine cancer, and ovarian cancer. It can be seen that the incidence of cancer is not the same in different sex groups in China. In order to achieve better results, we need to consider the gender differences in the dissemination of cancer medical knowledge. Taking age as an example, people's health concerns and demands are not the same throughout their life. For example, perimenopause is the performance of women's ovarian function decline and their reproductive function tends to terminate. Women in this stage, due to the decrease of estrogen secretion, will have a series of symptoms with autonomic nervous system dysfunction and neuropsychological symptoms, which are called perimenopausal syndrome, also known as menopausal syndrome. At the same time, osteoporosis is very easy to occur. Therefore, women at this stage will pay more attention to menopausal syndrome, postmenopausal osteoporosis, and other topics. But for young women, because they are far away from menopause, they are less likely to pay attention to such topics, and may pay more attention to the medical knowledge of childbearing, reproductive health, and parenting. So, we should pay attention to choosing different topics in different age groups to meet their health needs in medical communication. Taking life habits as an example, while cooking, Ningbo people tend to add much salt in general, and their salt intake may exceed the standard. At the same time, Ningbo people like to eat a lot of salted food, which has a high content of nitrosamines. And long-term consumption of it may cause cancer. However, Suzhou people's cooking is generally sweet and their sugar intake is high. So when we popularize healthy diet for these two people with different living habits, we should consider their different eating habits and popularize them with goals. Generally speaking, for the context of residents' health issues, we need to consider various factors such as region, age, gender, living habits, folk culture, and try to fit their different health demands, so as to maximize and optimize the effect of medical communication.

Finally, medical health issues are closely related to everyone, so medical communicators should also let the public participate in the discussion and dialogue of medical affairs, and actively establish a democratic mechanism in the field of medical decision-making. At the same time, the public should play an important role in the decision-making of medical communication. For example, during the Spring Festival of 2018, an article entitled "Beijing middle age under the flu" was widely circulated on social media. The author is an ordinary middle-class citizen living in Beijing. In this article, the author described the whole process of 29 days of medical treatment from the pneumonia caused by influenza to the death of his father-in-law. This article written by an ordinary person, including tens of thousands of words, should be said that was too long for online articles, and usually few people would read it all. However, in a few days, this long article had been read by hundreds of thousands or even millions of people and had aroused wide discussion, because his identity and narration fit the common sense and concerns of most ordinary people. In the eyes of professionals, this article may have various misconceptions in medicine. But after careful analysis, first of all, he raised a topic that people were most concerned about in the season of influenza epidemic in China in the last winter and this spring. It is about the medical and health problems that the public paid most attention to at that time. Secondly, he described a seemingly simple medical problem that eventually led to death from the perspective of ordinary people, which is more in line with the thinking of ordinary people in that condition. Many people will have a feeling of empathy after reading this article. This article not only aroused wide public resonance, but also inspired medical communicators to create a series of popular science articles to popularize influenza prevention measures, and targeted questions and answers, and achieved good popular science results, which played a positive role in the final control of influenza to a certain extent.

3. Relationship between medical communication and medical research

For various reasons, the majority of scientific workers have largely ignored the work of science popularization, and even there is a common misunderstanding that the work of science popularization will cause a waste of time and energy for scientific research. In fact, science popularization can effectively supplement scientific research and bring positive effects.

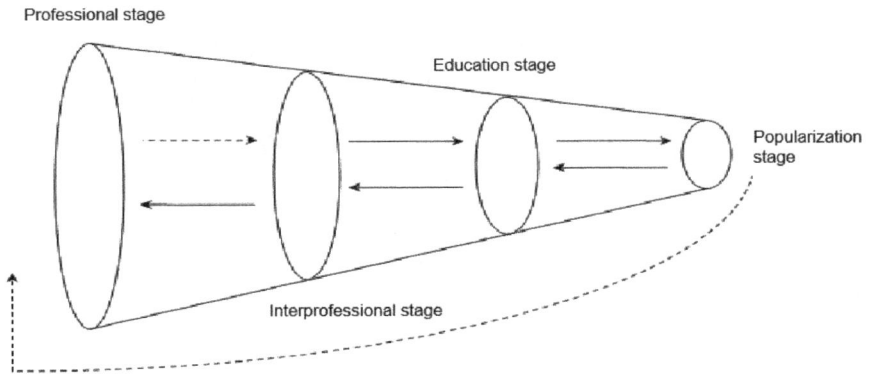

Figure 2.3   The continuum model of science communication.

The continuum model of science communication by Dr. Butch, a famous international science communication scientist, is used to explain the relationship between scientific research and science popularization (Figure 2.3).

The model divides scientific knowledge into four stages. The first level is the intraspecialistic stage, which refers to the knowledge accumulation and exchange within the discipline domain. Because the people who master the knowledge in this stage are experts and scholars in this field, they have and can spread the most knowledge. For example, the orthopedic knowledge that orthopedic doctors can communicate with each other is the most abundant, because they have the same discipline terminology. The second stage is the interspecialistic stage. Although they are both scientists, the range of communication between experts in different disciplines is narrowed than that of the first stage. For example, when orthopedic doctors communicate with physicians, the scope of communication is much smaller. The third is the educational stage. The knowledge suitable for teaching in textbooks in each scientific field is only a limited part of the subject field, usually which have been tested by time, while the most cutting-edge and up-to-date knowledge is not suitable for this level. For example, on July 25, 1978, Louise Brown, the world's first test tube baby, was born successfully in the UK. The success of this small life was hailed as a "miracle" by the media. The scientists had been experimenting for ten years without success until Louise was born. It should be said that Louise's birth ushered in a new era. It meant that many infertile families have the hope of bearing offspring. But in the 1970s and 1980s, when the IVF technology was just invented, it didn't test by time. Whether technology itself would do short-term or long-term harm to the mother, whether babies born with the help of technology were like ordinary babies, whether they would die, whether there would be various health or intellectual problems, including ethical problems, which could not be solved when the technology just came into being, so it was not suitable to appear in textbooks. But now, 40 years later, it has been proved to be a very effective method of assisted reproduction, and the offspring it produced has also been proved to be healthy. Louise, the first test tube baby, is now a mother herself. Robert Edwards, the founder of technology, won the Nobel Prize for physiology and medicine. This technology has been proven not only effective but also safe. It brings hope to millions of families who have lost the hope of future generations, and has been widely written into textbooks. The last is the popular stage, at which the amount of knowledge is the least, because the knowledge suitable for the public to popularize should have its choice gold standard, which is the scientific knowledge with final conclusion, including the contents of current science textbooks, dictionaries, and relevant national laws and regulations. For example, on November 13, 2017, at the annual meeting of the American Heart Association (AHA), the latest version of *The Guidelines for Prevention, Testing, Evaluation and Management of Hypertension in the United States* was released, jointly developed by AHA, the American Heart Association (ACC), and other academic institutions. The guideline has changed the standard of hypertension for many years: systolic blood pressure ≥ 140 and/or diastolic blood pressure ≥ 90 mmHg, redefined the new standard of hypertension, and put forward that systolic blood pressure ≥ 130 and/or diastolic blood pressure ≥ 80 mmHg can be diagnosed as hypertension. Since the standard of hypertension, which has been used for many years, has been redefined, the guideline has been controversial since it was issued. Some people think that the new standard of hypertension is lower than before, reflecting the importance of early intervention in hypertension. When the blood pressure is ≥ 130/80 mmHg, the intervention can avoid more complications of hypertension and target organ damage, which is beneficial to patients. It is also believed that the standard revision of the new guidelines is driven by economic interests, that is to say the new guidelines can drive manufacturers to sell more high blood pressure drugs. It is also believed that the new guidelines may increase the medical expenses of patients and the adverse reactions of drugs. On the other hand, they are not suitable for all patients with hypertension. Low blood pressure may also bring additional risks to patients. From the perspective of medical communication, our textbook and the recognized gold standard for the diagnosis of hypertension are always blood pressure $\geq$ 140/90 mmHg. The latest guidelines have not been widely recognized and are still in the stage of controversy. At present, when we do medical communication, we should use the latter (the textbook standard) rather than the former (the latest guide, which has not been widely recognized) as the standard to spread and popularize. Of course, if the new standard has been widely proved to be reliable and effective several years later, and has been written into textbooks, and the general public has also recognized the new standard of hypertension, the new standard should prevail in the dissemination of knowledge about hypertension at that time.

The above-mentioned stages are not independent. They can promote and influence each other. Even the popularized knowledge can also feed back to the professional field.

In the field of medicine, medical communication and medical research can form a closed-loop. Science popularization can be done according to the problems and conclusions found in scientific research, and scientific research can be guided by the effect and feedback of science popularization. The visibility of research can be effectively improved at the same time.

For example, *New York Times* is a daily newspaper published in New York, the United States. It is distributed all over the world and has a huge influence. The representatives of American high-level newspapers and serious journals have a good credibility and authority for a long time. *The New England Journal of Medicine*, one of the top medical journal, pointed out that a medical research article reported by the *New York Times* would be cited three times as frequently as other articles not reported by it.[6]

---

[6] Phillips, D. M. (1991). Importance of the lay press in the transmission of medical knowledge to the scientific community. *New England Journal of Medicine, 10,* 1180–1183.

4. Case analysis

Medical communication is mainly aimed at the general public without medical knowledge, who are also known as the common people. Therefore, scientificity and accuracy are very important, otherwise it will mislead the common people. In the last section, we mentioned that the knowledge suitable for popularization to the public should have a gold standard in the stage of popularization of scientific knowledge. The scientific knowledge must have a conclusion. However, there are some medical staff who neglect to do medical science popularization and medical communication, and think that doing medical science popularization and medical communication is just making a fuss, out of business and a waste of time. In fact, this is a misunderstanding of the concept.

Medical communication, medical research, and academic fields complement each other and interact well. Science popularization mainly focuses on the needs of the public. The topics are from academic research. At the same time, science popularization also needs to learn from academic achievements, lift academic status, and produce topics of scientific research while conducting science popularization. Scientific research further improves science popularization at the same time. We analyze a specific case. For example, among the fracture patients over 50 years old in the orthopedic ward of a hospital, doctors found that many of them were brittle fracture, which is the fracture occurred without trauma or slight trauma, and most of them were diagnosed of osteoporosis through further examination. Osteoporosis is a group of bone diseases caused by many reasons. Bone tissue has normal calcification. Calcium salt is in normal proportion to matrix. The metabolic bone disease is characterized by the decrease of bone tissue in unit volume. In most osteoporosis, the decrease of bone tissue is mainly due to the increase of bone absorption. Osteoporosis is usually characterized by bone pain and easy fracture. With the above findings, doctors conducted a survey of osteoporosis knowledge among people over 50 years old, and found that many people are concerned about osteoporosis, but it is not clear what kind of people will get osteoporosis, what symptoms and hazards of osteoporosis, and how to prevent and treat osteoporosis. It is a good topic to carry out science popularization or medical communication about osteoporosis for

people over 50 years old, which can be seen as a typical science popularization topic found in academic activities. How shall we do the science
popularization of osteoporosis then? The audience of popular science is
ordinary people, who have no medical knowledge, so the content popularized must be scientific and accurate, and the opinions must have exact
basis. This means that communicators have to look up a lot of documents
and materials, especially textbooks, in order to complete a scientific
popularization with a sound basis and a correct viewpoint. This is what
science popularization should learn from academic. The rigorous attitude
required for learning science is extremely important. The preciseness of
science popularization is also vital. It must not be cursory, otherwise it
may bring confusion or even harm to the general public. In the process of
popularizing osteoporosis among the above-mentioned people, besides
orthopedic doctors, other relevant departments, such as osteoporosis doctors, nutrition doctors, clinical pharmacists, rehabilitation doctors, and
nursing personnel, are invited to participate in the process. This not only
facilitates the audience but also enables them to receive the required
knowledge of osteoporosis at the same time. Medical knowledge, including nutrition, medicine, nursing, rehabilitation, and other links, also drives
the common development of these other related departments and orthopedics, forming a multi-disciplinary cooperation of medical communication
and science popularization. Then in order to reduce the incidence of brittle fracture and the rate of refracture in the high-risk group, we need to
intervene the fracture group and the high-risk group. During the intervention, other relevant hospitals and community health service centers were
invited to carry out the intervention of high-risk factors. In addition to the
hospital, primary health care institutions such as lower level hospitals or
community health service centers are also promoted, forming a mechanism of up-down linkage and joint participation, and may eventually build
a bone health communication base that affects the whole region. The
radiation and benefited population will continue to expand. Then, in the
process of bone health transmission, we need to evaluate the effect of
fracture patients and general high-risk groups, respectively. At this time,
if a health evaluation system is established for these two groups, and the
effect of the health system is evaluated respectively, and the incidence of
brittle fracture and the incidence of refracture of patients with brittle

fracture in high-risk groups are evaluated at the same time, which is the problem of scientific research found in the popular science. While evaluating the health system's effect on these people, scientific research can further improve the effect of science popularization (Figure 2.4). Therefore, it can be seen that scientific research and popular science can complement each other and develop together.

For example, the incidence of liver cancer in a certain place is relatively high. Through epidemiological investigation, it is found that local residents like to eat salted food, and salted food contains nitrosamine, which has been widely recognized as a strong carcinogen, also as one of the most important chemical carcinogens. Long-term consumption may induce gastrointestinal cancer. According to the incidence of local diseases and the results of flow regulation, science popularization about eating less salted food and preventing liver cancer is a science popularization topic found by the academic, which can well meet the needs of local residents. After actively popularizing science among the local population, long-term follow-up survey was carried out to assess whether the incidence of liver cancer in the local area had declined, which is a good scientific research topic derived from popular science. Such an organic combination of complementary scientific research and popular science may improve the diet of local residents and then reduce the incidence of liver cancer. Ultimately disease prevention and control are achieved, in line with the current concept of prevention first and healthy China, and real benefits are brought to the people.

When choosing the topic of medical communication, we also need to pay attention to the needs of people and do some academic research, to understand what people's most missing knowledge or basic needs are. People with the same disease may have different missing parts or needs. If we can carry out targeted science popularization for different needs, we can get twice the result with half the effort. For example, hypertension is a very common chronic disease, which is characterized by high blood pressure of systemic circulation artery. It can damage many target organs, such as heart, brain, kidney, etc., and even cause death or disability. In 2017, the "12th Five-Year Plan" sampling survey was announced at the China heart conference; it was to study 500,000 residents over 15 years old in 31 provinces and cities in China. It shows that the prevalence of

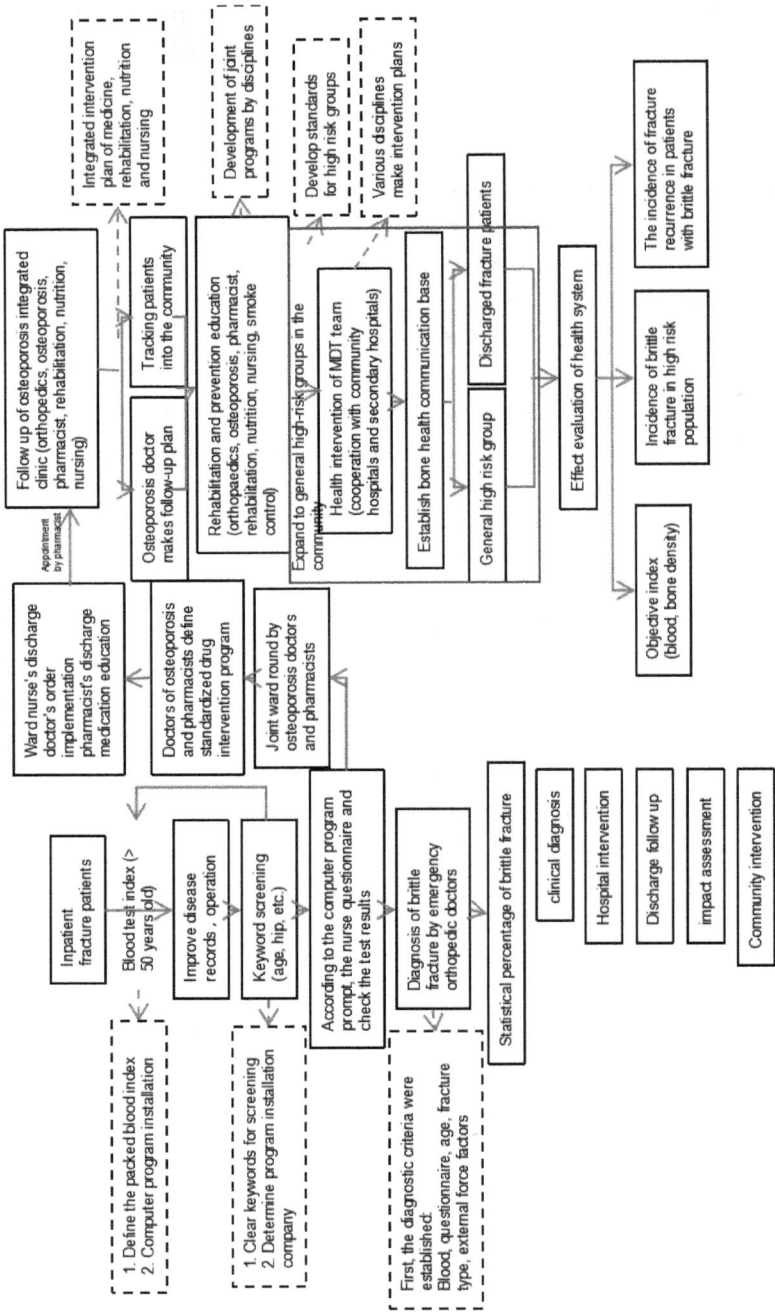

Figure 2.4   Relationship between osteoporosis research and science popularization.

hypertension is 23%, which means that about one out of every four people is a patient with hypertension. The prevalence of hypertension reaches 243.5 million, while the prevalence of normal high blood pressure is 436.3 million. However, the awareness rate of hypertension is only 42.7%, and the control rate is only 14.5%, which means that less than half of the people know about hypertension. On average, only 1.5 of the 10 hypertensive patients have reached the standard of blood pressure control. The survey also shows that the difference between urban and rural areas in the prevalence of hypertension is narrowing, and there is no significant difference between urban and rural people in the prevalence of hypertension, but the awareness rate and treatment of hypertension are lower and less in rural areas. At this time, if carrying out academic research on hypertension in urban and rural areas respectively, we will find that the reasons for the high incidence and low control rate of hypertension in urban and rural populations are not the same. The high incidence and low control rate of hypertension in urban population may be due to high work pressure, long-term high tension in the mental state, unhealthy living and eating habits, lack of necessary sports, misleading by incorrect information through frequent internet search, lack of time for medical treatment, failure to see a doctor correctly, failure to regular treatment, poor treatment compliance, etc. However, the high incidence and low control rate of rural population are more likely due to the factors of low educational level, lack of awareness of the importance of hypertension, low economic income, heavy medical burden, difficult access to medical resources, relatively difficult access to medical services, relatively lack of medical care, lack of family company, etc. Then, according to the results of the survey, to urban and rural populations of two different kinds, carrying out more targeted medical communication and popular science for their own reasons will have good results.

In the regional survey of hypertension, it was found that Beijing (35.9%), Tianjin (34.5%), and Shanghai (29.1%) ranked in the top three cities in China, followed by Liaoning, Yunnan, Guangdong, and Heilongjiang, which belonged to the first echelon; Jilin, Shanxi, Jiangsu, Tibet, Hanan, Fujian, Sichuan, Guizhou, Hebei, Zhejiang, and other provinces had relatively low prevalence, belonging to the second. The prevalence of hypertension was 15.6% in Hunan Province. According to the results of the regional survey, the prevalence of hypertension in the first echelon areas is in urgent need of the related knowledge, and the second and third echelons also need to be paid enough attention. In the past survey of hypertension, the prevalence of hypertension in China has always shown a feature of "high in the north and low in the south". The academic circles think that it may be related to people in the north eating more salt. However, in this survey, it is found that the feature of "high in the north and low in the south" has been weakened. Maybe because of the wide-range communication and interaction among regions, the northern restaurants have opened in the south, and southern dishes are also distributed in the north, and the difference in diet between the north and the south is gradually narrowing. People in the south are eating more and more salty food now, which increases the prevalence of hypertension, and the phenomenon of high in the north and low in the south is gradually decreasing. Even in regions with similar prevalence, further research can also find that their high prevalence may have different characteristics and factors. For example, in some places, the high prevalence of hypertension is due to the local diet structure dominated by high salt diet, while in some places, the high prevalence is due to high oil and high fat diet. Then, for people in these two different regions, science popularization with different emphasis on improving the diet structure has achieved the goal of focusing on the needs of the people. In the meantime, the selection of topics comes from academic research; thus the effect will be better than science popularization without emphasis. The ultimate goal of science popularization and medical communication is to reduce the morbidity and mortality of diseases, to improve people's health level, and to realize the ideal of healthy urban area and healthy China. Only when people's health is guaranteed can the country develop better.

Part II

Doctor–Patient Communication: Medical Communication in the Clinic

Chapter 3

Basic Models and Characteristics of Doctor–Patient Communication

1. Medical models

1.1. *Introduction*

"Model" is a concept in mathematical logic, serving as a formula expressing the theory of formal logic. Later, "model" went beyond mathematical logic and was extensively used in natural science and social science to summarize the core world outlooks and methodologies of each discipline. Medical model, namely medical viewpoint, is man's generalization of the nature of medicine in the course of medical practice in his struggle against diseases. Medical model not only comprises the basic characteristics of medicine, but also indicates the basic concept of medical practice.[1] In the history of mankind, medical model underwent a number of transformations with the progress of science and technology and the cognitive development of man's own life processes.[2] Before doing the practice of medical communication, it is necessary to learn various medical models.

---

[1] Wang, J. (2006). *Physician–patient communication*. Beijing: People's Medical Publishing House.

[2] Zhao, S. (2010). *Public relations in hospitals*. Beijing: Science Press.

1.2. *Five different models*

1.2.1. *Model 1: Spiritual medical model*

Spiritual medical model originated in ancient times when productivity was low; humans began to observe the phenomena of life and think about the essence of disease and health. However, humans' perception of the world at that time was limited by direct observation, which made them fail to interpret wind and rain, thunder and lightning, earthquake, tsunami, and other natural phenomena with scientific viewpoints; as a result, their understanding of life was also supernatural. They believed there were great supernatural powers ruling the world, which brought about the formation of the primitive religious concept of "god", and brought about religious activities such as prayer and divination. Ancient humans believed life and health were given by god; diseases and disasters were caused by the wrath of heaven or possession of ghosts; death resulted from the gods recalling human souls. Therefore, the treatment of diseases and preservation of health in those days principally relied on praying to gods, divining by the Eight Diagrams, and asking gods for forgiveness, and so on. The principal methods for treatment included induced emesis and diarrhea accompanied by the application of some plants- and minerals-based medicines. According to the spiritual medical model, witchcraft and medicine were always intertwined with each other. Despite a primitive medical model, it has a certain influence in some remote areas and on certain populations in the world today.

The outlook on disease as per the spiritual medical model is considered an ontological view of disease. According to such view, the causes of diseases were entities that existed independently of the human body, and its relationship with the human body was between entities. One of the important forms of such ontological outlook on disease was that patients acquired something alien from the outside and that the diseases were the work of such alien things in the human body. In a variety of ways, ancient people imagined how such alien things were acquired from the outside world. Another important form of the ontological outlook on disease as per the spiritual medical model was to believe diseases were caused by the loss of soul, a vital factor of their lives. The soul lived in healthy people and gave them life, "having mastered the thought and speech of their lives". However, once "soul" was lost, people may get sick or die. Similarly, the reasons why patients lost their lives were also imagined in various manners: Patients may get frightened, which "drove away" the warm soul; someone may put a soul trap in the path of a patient; alternatively, the soul was "taken away" by a wizard or devil; and so on. The mystery of outlook on disease based on the spiritual medical model determines the mystery of its being used for disease treatment. Their treatment techniques were mysterious. This is embodied by "exorcism" and "evocation", the two methods of treatment corresponding to the two forms of spiritual ontology outlook on disease.

Let me give you an example for interpreting the spiritual medical model. For instance, if someone became delirious, foaming at the mouth, spasmodic, and aphasic, which is to say, he failed to move and speak all of a sudden, the patient is likely to have had a stroke (apoplexy) from the modern scientific medical perspective; but in ancient times when the medical level was far less developed than today, the causes of many diseases were unrevealed, so people at the time probably thought such patient was "bewitched", that is, the evil spirit's penetration or possession by devil resulted in his obnubilation and hemiplegia; in such a case, people would call a witch physician or a master to exorcise the patient, since they firmly believed that exorcism would restore the patient's health and vitality; if exorcism did not work, it might be because the patient was so deeply bewitched that even gods could not save him. This is an example of the ancient application of spiritual medical model, although the spiritual medical model seems a little ridiculous or superstitious today. It neither revealed the essence of human diseases, nor provided people with effective and scientific methods to cure diseases; however, as the first structured medical system in human history, it preserved and spread the medical experience of primitive humans, and created conditions for the birth of ancient medicine to some extent, having encouraged and invigorated the primitive humans to triumph over illness. Under the very limited form of knowledge or practice in ancient times, it might be the most appropriate medical model; moreover, it is also an indispensable part in the continuous progress of human medical model.

1.2.2. *Model 2: Nature philosophical medical model*

Religion is the result of the submission to and the mystification of the forces of nature, while medicine is the result of conquering and clarifying the forces of nature. With the development of productivity and living standard, people came to know a variety of natural phenomena and tried to interpret the etiology and pathogenesis of diseases from a natural point of view; additionally, they gathered extensive experience in treatment of diseases with animals, plants, and minerals that offering pharmacological effects; thus, it's an empirical medical model. The origins of Chinese and Western medicine involved dialectics of nature and naive materialism, which gave birth to the nature philosophical medical model. The ancient Chinese medicine comprises pathological theories such as "the yin-yang and the five elements", "the six evils (external factors)" (i.e., wind evil, cold evil, summer-heat evil, damp evil, dryness evil, fire evil), and "the seven emotions (internal factors)" (i.e., happy, angry, anxious, missing, sad, scared, and frightened). According to the theory of yin-yang and the five elements, Yin and Yang mutually reinforce, neutralize, and inhibit each other, while the internal organs of human body maintain a balance; once the normal balance is broken, diseases may occur; the disease in one organ may cause others to get damaged. The six evils are associated with and different from the six factors in nature. Under normal circumstances, "wind, cold, summer heat, wetness, dryness, and fire" represent the six different kinds of climate change in the world of nature, which are collectively called "the six factors in nature". The constant change in the six factors in nature determines the climatic change, namely "spring wind, summer heat (fire), autumn dryness, winter cold, and long summer wetness". The human body is adaptable to the six factors in nature through self-regulation, so such factors normally cause no diseases to the human body. When the climate change goes beyond a certain limit, for instance, in the event of the excess or inadequacy of the six factors in nature, the incorrect timing of energy (e.g. cold spring or hot autumn, etc.), and the sudden change of climate (e.g. sharp temperature reduction or fierce rise of temperature, etc.), to which the human body fails to get adapted, diseases may frequently occur; in the case of insufficient anti-pathogenic energy and weakened immunity, the wind evil, cold evil, summer-heat evil, damp evil, dryness evil, and fire evil may invade the body and lead to diseases; in such a case, the six factors in nature are referred to as "the six evils". Since the six evils are unhealthy factors, they are also known as "the six exopathogens". Therefore, the definition of the six factors in nature/the six evils is dependent on whether diseases come on or not. According to the theory of seven emotions, "the seven emotions" refer to the seven emotional activities of the human body, and the different mental states caused by various external stimuli; the emotional changes caused by external environment are induced by the physiological activities of the five internal organs, so the seven emotions are called "five expressions of emotions" that connect respectively to the five internal organs; excessive "seven emotions" are defined as mental pathogenic factors, which may cause immediate damage to the corresponding internal organs. Ancient Greek medical experts believed life was made up of water, fire, air, and earth, which worked respectively with cold, hot, dry, and wet substances to constitute the four liquids of human body, that is, the blood, yellow bile, black bile, and mucus; the different proportions of the four body fluids in the human body bring about different temperaments; short-tempered and quick-acting people have "bilious temperament"; active and flexibly-acting people have "sanguineous temperament"; quiet and lumbering people have "phlegmatic temperament"; fragile and heavy-footed people have "melancholic temperament". Diseases are caused by the imbalance of the four fluids, which may result from external factors; therefore, the harmony and balance of the four body fluids determine the temperament and health of human body. Compared with spiritual medical model, the nature philosophical medical model links health and disease to the natural and social environments of human life to establish the view of human–environment integration, having thereby enlightened medicine and convincingly promoted the evolution of medicine.

Let's present some examples of nature philosophical medical model. According to the *Inner Canon of Huangdi*, the first medical book of ancient China written over 2000 years ago, "violent joy impairs the heart; anger damages the liver; melancholy impairs the lung; anxiety impairs the spleen; fear impairs the kidney". Violent emotions may result in the dysfunction of Yin–Yang balance in the internal organs and the energy–blood circulation disorder. When we say "violent joy impairs the heart", we mean too much joy spoils the state of mind; TCM holds that "the heart controls mental activities". The heart is the center of emotional thinking activities, while joy is the expression of a happy mood; joy contributes to smooth energy-blood circulation and muscular relaxation, helping remove physical fatigue. As the saying goes, "joy puts heart into a man"; something cheerful makes people in high spirits, but excessive joy may cause damage to the state of mind — this is exactly what the wording "extreme joy begets sorrow" means; "anger damaging the liver" means long-term suppressed indignation may bring about hepatic depression syndrome; TCM holds that liver energy should be free and smooth; tender liver makes blood harmonious, while the stagnation of liver brings about circulation of vital energy in the wrong direction. Anger is a common emotion; rage causes energy to flow upwards, which causes the liver to fail to act freely; this may lead to transverse dysfunction of liver energy: For instance, some people, after losing their temper, often develop hypochondriac pain or fullness below their ribs; TCM describes this phenomenon as "transverse invasion of the hyperactive liver-energy offends the spleen". When we say "melancholy impairs the lung", we mean the depression of liver energy and the dissipation of energy-Yin occur in sad and anxious people. TCM holds that anxiety is a sentiment closely connected with the lung, and sadness may impair the lung, thereby leading to shortness of breath, dry cough, hemoptysis and hoarseness, and so on; as the further development of anxiety, sorrow is a mood caused by sadness and goes as pale complexion and inadequate vitality. Since both anxiety and sorrow impair the lung, so people believe "too much sorrow impairs the lung and energy diabetes when the lungs are damaged". When it comes to the wording "anxiety impairs the spleen", it means worry beyond measure may result in spleen energy stagnation; the healthy energy will be impaired and abnormal transportation and transformation may happen if this lasts long. TCM holds that "contemplation causes energy stagnation"; worry beyond measure may bring about the dysfunction of the nervous system and the decreased secretion of digestive juices, which may lead to loss of appetite, insomnia and dreamful sleep, neurasthenia, and so on, which have certain connection with the spleen. "Fear impairing the kidney" means that fear may impair kidney energy; the timidity caused by excessive mental stress may lead to urinary incontinence, spermatorrhea and other symptoms; being frightened refers to the mental stress resulting from sudden change in things. TCM holds that the kidney stores the essence and affects the reproductive system, which is to say, kidneys are engines of life; ancient physicians called the kidneys as "congenital foundation"; a person who gets stunned and pinned by sudden fright may feel ill at ease, which may arise from the reversed circulation of heart energy and the impaired blood. It should be noted that the physicians of TCM in those days have found that normal emotional activities were different reactions of physical and psychological activities of the human body to stimuli from the external environment; as emotional experiences that every people had, normal emotional activities usually did not cause or induce diseases. However, intense and persistent emotional stimulation that goes beyond the physiological and psychological adaptation of human body may cause damage to the internal organs and vital essence, which may lead to dysfunction, weak vital energy of human body or vital essence deficiency of internal organs; the resulting poor ability to adapt to emotional stimulation may cause or induce diseases, which are commonly known as "internal injuries caused by seven emotions". For example, according to the short fiction *Fan Jin Passed Provincial Civil Service Examination*, Fan Jin's suddenly passing the provincial exam in his old age caused him to be too excited (since he failed many exams before), thus developing violent superexcitation and the disorder of mind, which demonstrates how "violent joy impairs the heart". In *The Romance of the Three Kingdoms*, Zhuge Liang with superior wisdom enraged Zhou Yu, a great general of the Kingdom of Wu, to death, which demonstrates how "anger damages the liver". In *A Dream in Red Mansions*, Lin Daiyu died of lung disease caused by long-term depression, which typically demonstrates how "melancholy impairs the lung". The long-term worry beyond measure resulting from some things that happen in life may bring about insomnia, which representatively demonstrates how "anxiety impairs the spleen". As the saying goes, "someone is shit scared"; when a person is excessively afraid, his kidney energy dissipates, and the resulting poor consolidation at the kidneys may lead to incontinence. When compared with spiritual medical model, the nature philosophical medical model revealed the etiology and mechanism of some diseases in an imperfect manner; however, it was quite an accomplishment in view of the undeveloped medical conditions then and represents a great advance in the history of medicine based on certain scientific basis and reasons even from the perspective of modern medicine.

1.2.3. *Model 3: Mechanistic medical model*

Since the Renaissance in the 16th century, the metaphysical mechanical materialism-based view of nature that explains all natural phenomena by "forces" and "mechanical motions" has been developed with the establishment of Newton's theory system of classical mechanics. The mechanistic model of medicine was born during the Renaissance that spanned the 14th, 15th, and 16th centuries. In the critique of scholasticism, the mechanical materialism replaced the idealist view of life and medicine, having created conditions for the rise of modern experimental medicine. Bacon, a British natural scientist and philosopher, presented an idea of "studying nature experimentally" and advocated the study of anatomy and pathological anatomy. Descartes, a French philosopher clearly presented his point of view that "organisms are nothing more than sophisticated machines", according to which, the physiological movement of organisms was simply concluded as physical and chemical changes, and even mental activities were considered mechanical motions. During that period, the representative works of mechanistic medical model included *Animals Are Machines* (by Descartes) and *L'homme-Machine* (by La Mettrie, a French physician and philosopher). Descartes held that the difference between human and animal lied in that the former had soul, while the latter did not. Hence, the behavior of animals was completely subject to the laws of mechanical motion. As far as human was concerned, the activity of human body was also subject to the laws of mechanical motion apart from the soul. In that way, enlightened by Harvey's mechanistic explanation of blood circulation, Descartes thought of animals and humans as automatic machines based on the principles of mechanics and anatomical experiments from the perspective of the mechanical principles of physics. He believed that one end of the thin line in neural tube was connected to sensory organs while the other was connected to the openings of certain passages in the brain; when a sensory organ was stimulated by external objects, such fine line would be pulled, and the piston opening of pore passage would thus be opened; then, the animal spirit in ventricle would drive other substances in ventricle from the brain into the muscles; when a certain extent is reached, the muscles would be inflated to bring about motions. This is the first description of reflex action and its physiological mechanism, reflex arc, in the human history. La Mettrie affirmed Descartes' describing the animals only for material reasons, but he disagreed Descartes' seeing animals as simple automata without sensory capacity. La Mettrie advocated defining humans as sensible living machines with spirit and believed that the conditions of human body determined the conditions of mind all the time, and that the human tissues were automata like clocks, which were totally governed by the mechanical laws of material. La Mettrie demonstrated the dependence of the mind on tissues, especially on human brain based on the wealth of scientific data on medicine, physiology, and anatomy available. Going further than Descartes, he saw the brain as the seat of the mind or soul.

Under the mechanistic medical model, medicine made great progress. British physician Harvey discovered blood circulation; in *An Anatomical Study of the Motion of the Heart and of the Blood in Animals*, a book he published in 1628, Harvey systematically summarized the law of blood circulation he discovered and its experimental basis. That 72-page book is a landmark in the history of physiology. It is Harvey's historic exploit that the blood circulation was discovered on the basis of previous work; he brought the experimental method into biology through the discovery of blood circulation. Morgagni, an Italian pathologist published *On the Location and Cause of the Disease*; based on 640 anatomical cases, he believed that disease was a local damage and that every disease could be traced to a corresponding lesion in an organ. Morgagni clearly demonstrated that normal anatomy was the basis of pathological anatomy, and linked the phenomenon of disease and the pathological changes organically, arguing that organs were locations of diseases and organ changes were the cause of diseases; furthermore, he established the theory of organ pathology and defined the new concept of disease.

The mechanistic medical model brought medicine into the era of experimental medicine and made outstanding contributions to the progress and development of medicine. However, the mechanistic medical model has its historical deficiency by reason that it thinks of human beings as machines and deals with too one-sided observation of the human body by neglecting the biological complexity and effects of social environment and the social attributes and biological properties of humans. It should be noted that mechanistic medical ideology exhibits duality for the development of medicine. On the one hand, it holds that human body is absolutely mechanical, thereby excluding the effects of biological, psychological, and social factors on health and frequently explaining biological phenomena in terms of physical and chemical concepts; on the other hand, the mechanistic theory brought about real progress in anatomy and biology, having greatly promoted the evolution of medical science.

For instance, if we compare the human body to a car, the heart should be the engine; the car can be started again by simply replacing the broken engine, but if someone has a heart problem, will the replacement of the heart work? The answer is no. On the one hand, every human is a whole, rather than a machine that can be disassembled at will; if the heart goes wrong, other organs may go wrong, too, so a replacement heart alone won't solve all the organ problems. On the other hand, since heart sources are extremely scarce, the replacement of heart is an arduous task; even if the heart can be successfully changed, nobody can guarantee that the patient's personality will not change, that his/her daily living capability can be fully recovered, that his/her cardiac function can be restored, that his/her psychological enduring capacity is acceptable, and that he/she can return to the community and work like a normal person. The patients' capacity of daily physical, psychological, and social activities may need to be reassessed, and the patients may need some help. Thus it can be seen that humans are not simple machines, and medical treatment is not a matter of part replacement; these are the limitations of mechanistic medical model.

1.2.4. *Model 4: Biomedical model*

By publishing the book *Motion of the Heart and Blood* in 1628, British physician Harvey established his blood circulation theory as the beginning of modern medicine; many great achievements and discoveries were made in the biological science in this period. Morgagni's the study of organ localization of disease and Virchow from Germany systematically discussed the theory of cytopathology, and emphasized that "all cells are derived from previous cells" and all diseases were cellular diseases, thereby breaking with the dominant humoral pathology at that time, having greatly advanced the development of pathology; the resulting immeasurable impact on the diagnosis and treatment of diseases and the establishment of cytopathology of epoch-making significance and so on have laid the foundation of modern medicine. The medical science in this period was based on biological science and began to form a biomedical model. The three discoveries of natural science in the 19th century, that is, the law of conservation of energy, the cell theory, and the evolutionism, further promoted the development of biology and medicine, and scientific methods were extensively used in medical practice; in those days, the awareness of health was greatly improved, and the biomedical concept of health was established.

Based on biological science, the biomedical model is focused on the relations and laws among etiology, host, and natural environment. Biological technologies mushroomed with the industrial revolution and began to challenge infectious diseases. The epidemic of cholera and typhoid in the 1840s urged Pasteur, a French scientist and Koch, a German microbiologist and other scientists to systematically study bacteria, which set the foundation for bacteriological theory of etiology; the cytopathological theory established by Virchow pushed people's understanding of disease into the cellular stage. The world gained a new understanding of health and disease: Health is the result of preserving the dynamic balance among the host, environment, and pathogen, while illness is the result of the loss of such balance. The biomedical model turned into the foundation of medical experimental research, having promoted the scientific and systematic researches on human physiological activities and diseases. Through sterilization and disinfestation, vaccination, and application of antibacterial drugs, humans won their first great victory in the field of public health by significantly reducing the incidence of acute and chronic infectious and parasitic diseases and remarkably improving the average life expectancy of human beings. In the meantime, the establishment of such basic medical sciences as physiology, anatomy, histology, embryology, and genetics provided a scientific basis for solving major problems in front of clinical medicine and preventive medicine, having pushed the evolution of the entire medicine from empiricism to scientism.

Let's take a simple example. For instance, a patient with hypertension developed acute myocardial infarction, the most serious heart disease; examination indicated that the patient's coronary stenosis ratio was 95%; fortunately, the patient survived after active rescue treatment. From the perspective of biomedical model, the major pathogeny of that patient was the vascular stenosis and occlusion resulting from the coronary athero-sclerotic plaques induced by hypertension; it was just necessary to place a stent in the narrow vessel, tell the patient to take hypertension drugs, antiplatelet drugs, and other adjuvant drugs on time; in fact, the patient got better after the placement of stent. Careful analysis indicated, however, that the patient's hypertension and heart disease were largely related to his psychological and social activities. He worked more than 10 hours a day under great pressure of work at a fast pace, which caused him to suffer from sleep insufficiency and has no time for exercise; moreover, he prac-ticed an unreasonable diet. In addition, the patient had a typical type A personality, which is to say, he was hot-tempered, loved to excel others, apt to be irritable, and constantly in the midst of anxiety. In the biomedical model alone, the treatment of hypertension and heart disease would be sufficient, but if his mental and social activities remain unchanged, it is likely that he will have similar diseases again in the near future.

In short, the biomedical model can be explained as follows: Cytopathic effect → Pathological changes of tissue structure → Dysfunction. Biomedical model represents a significant progress in medical develop-ment; studying the structure and function of organisms and their biologi-cal reactions to various internal and external environmental factors and disease processes is still a basic subject of medical research. However, this metaphysical way of learning "sees their existence without seeing their emergence, development and extinction, and sees their static state without remembering their motions". It should be noted that the biomedical model laid the foundation for experimental research, promoted the development of specific diagnostic and therapeutic methods, and made great contribu-tions to the control of infectious and parasitic diseases; however, it stressed "the centering on disease" without giving attention to the com-plexity of collective life and the influence of psychological, social, and environmental factors on human beings. In that model, disease seems to be an autonomous individual that can be explained by general criteria and has nothing to do with the patient's life background and social background; this thought is not true. As modern industrialization evolves, infectious diseases, parasitic diseases, and nutritional deficiencies are no longer major threats to human health, while the cardiovascular diseases, cerebrovascular diseases, cancer, public nuisance diseases, accidents and suicides, drug and alcohol abuse, overeating, and psychogenic diseases where psychological and social factors play an important role have become a major challenger to human health; diagnosis, treatment, and prevention of these diseases using biomedical models alone cannot solve the problems completely. While the mechanistic medical model regards man as a machine, the biomedical model analyzes and studies human diseases merely from a biological perspective with other factors ignored. However, man is a social animal, where the occurrence of the disease may also involve psychological and social factors; the biomedical model precisely overlooks this point, instead, it separates the patient from the disease, and normally performs isolated tests on tissue specimens from patients to search for pathogenic factors and find out the pathogens and key biological variables; instead of looking at a living person, it looks at body fluids and cells. Therefore, despite its important role in the fight against diseases, the biomedical model isolates humans from their social environment, loses sight of human sociality and subject consciousness, and neglects the human wholeness; moreover, its tendency to focus too much on technology and materialization makes it impossible to effectively solve the new problems in front of human beings today, and causes the lack of humanistic spirit; thus, a new model seems ready to come out.

1.2.5. *Model 5: Bio-psycho-social medical model*

After surviving terrible deadly diseases, humans begin to pursue longevity, balance of physical and mental pleasures, and harmonious social psychological atmosphere. However, the biomedical theory that focuses solely on individuals can't shoulder the responsibilities after the prevalence of many chronic noncommunicable diseases and various mental illnesses. The social health project involving all human beings pushed bio-psycho-social medical model onto the stage of history. This model was proposed in 1977 by Engel, a professor of psychiatry and internal medicine at the University of Rochester, the USA; according to Engel, the biomedical model exhibited the following shortcomings: "Diseases can be interpreted with measurable biological (somatic) variables deviating from normal; there is no room in its framework for the social, psychological and behavioral aspects of diseases"; in fact, biomedicine alone cannot solve the problems regarding the occurrence, prevalence, and prevention of diseases such as tuberculosis and sexually transmitted diseases, especially AIDS, and so on. AIDS and other sexually transmitted diseases are still out of control in countries with advanced biomedical technologies, because such diseases are more determined by people's lifestyles and behaviors, as well as such social factors as economic conditions and educational level. In the meantime, Bloom believed environment, heredity, behavior & lifestyle, and medical & health services were the four major factors that affected health; as the most important factors affecting health, the environmental factors included social and natural environmental factors; on this basis, he proposed the environment health medical model that placed emphasis on the impact of environmental factors, especially the social ones, on health. The comprehensive health medical model proposed by Lalonde and Dwyer further amended and supplemented the key factors affecting the diseases and health of the population, that is environmental factors, lifestyle and behavioral factors, biogenetic factors, and medical service factors. Since each of the four categories was composed of three factors, there were twelve factors in total. Various factors have different effects on different diseases; for instance, cerebrovascular diseases were principally associated with lifestyle and biological factors; accidental death was mainly caused by environmental factors; infectious diseases were closely associated with health services. According to Engel, to learn the determinants of diseases and achieve a rational model of treatment and health care, the medical model must take into account patients, the environments in which the patients live, and the complementary systems designed by society to cope with the destructive effects of diseases, namely the role of physicians and the health care system. Based on the principles of systems theory, Engel built the system framework of diseases, patients, and environments (natural and social environment). From atoms, molecules, cells, tissues, tissue systems to humans (whole), and then to the natural systems conceptualized and linked by humans, families, communities, and humans. The high-level coordination within and between systems is reflected in health; the restoration of health is the creation of a new coordination with a different system than before the occurrence of disease. All levels of the system affect each other, and any change at any level may affect the entire system, triggering the chain reaction in the system. Since this medical model recognizes the proper place of psychological and social factors in the medical research system, it exhibits important guiding significance in clinical medicine, preventive medicine, and public health services today.

The socialization of medical development enables the bio-psycho-social medical model to be the background for creation of modern medical model. Socialization of medical development refers to the process of transformation from individual decentralized medical activities to systematic medical activities performed based on social division of labor and collaboration. In this process, the responsibility for the health of residents lies not only with medical personnel, but also with the joint efforts of all sectors of the whole society. During the protection of human health and the fight against diseases, the limitations of individual activities are becoming increasingly apparent; only with the participation of the state and the society, as well as appropriate social measures, can we achieve favorable results. Under such a tendency, health care globalization and integration creep up. Secondly, the disease spectrum of modern society has changed, and the key components of human diseases have shifted from acute infectious diseases to chronic noncommunicable diseases; based on the change in disease spectrum, the "magic weapons" for treatment of diseases have also shifted from vaccination, sterilization and disinfestation, and antibacterial drugs to social medicine, behavioral medicine, and environmental medicine. Moreover, in this process, people's health concepts and needs are changing. Nowadays, people hope to get comprehensive and diversified medical and health services from treatment to prevention, from physical to psychological aspects, from inside to outside hospitals, as well as family care and community health care services; in the meantime, they begin to realize that diseases are not only caused by biological factors, but are also associated with such factors as diet, environment, and occupation. For the patient with myocardial infarction mentioned in the previous paragraph, the comprehensive embodiment of treatment with "bio-psycho-social medical model" should be as follows: During the treatment of hypertension and heart disease, physicians give attention to the high working and psychological stresses resulting from his unhealthy diets and living habits, interfere with his life and behavioral patterns, and relieve his working and psychological stresses; additionally, physicians provide certain psychological and social counseling for him to resume normal occupation after his illness, relieve his anxiety, and enable him to get adapted to his new job and life faster. During such a process, we not only treat diseases, but also cure the patient.

Emphasizing "centering on humans", the "bio-psycho-social medical model" (Figure 3.1) is established to prevent diseases and damages, promote and preserve health, relieve pain and suffering caused by illness, perform the treatment of disease and the care of the incurable diseases, avoid early death, and seek peaceful death. Humans have two fundamental attributes, that is naturality and sociality. First of all, humans have natural properties, and the cells, tissues, organs, and systems composed of natural materials constitute the microworld of human beings; additionally, humans are social; any human who exists in society has his/her specific backgrounds, including personal background, family background, social background, and so on; humans also have certain social connections, including their relations with others, the communities, the employers, and the states;

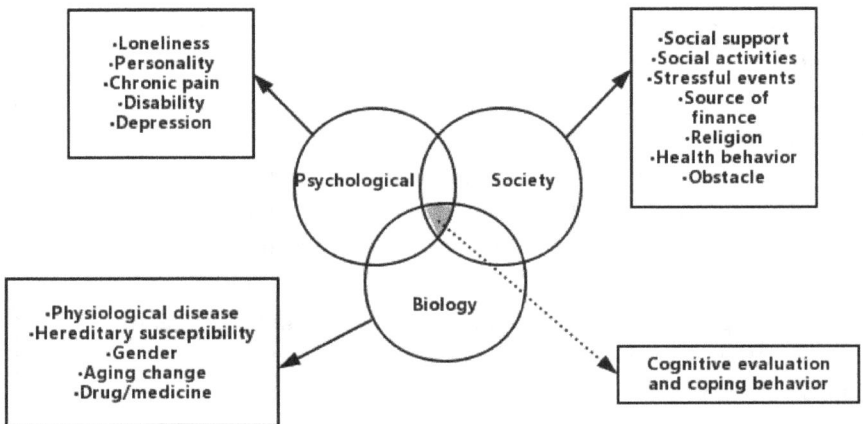

Figure 3.1 Bio-psycho-social medical model.

various backgrounds and relationships of human beings constitute the macroscopic world of social attributes. In the "bio-psycho-social medical model", medicine has to address the diseases, namely the microworld studied in the field of life science, and the macro world of humans studied in the fields of humanities and social sciences. From the perspective of microscopic world inside the system, each patient has disease attributes; but from the perspective of macro world, each patient is an individual with social and cultural backgrounds, and a person with independent personality; thus, medical personnel are required to provide him/her with "human-centered" health care. This model transforms the previous singular medical model of thinking into a comprehensive model of thinking, expands the territories of medical treatment and research, and promotes the disease prevention from purely physiological prevention to social and psychological prevention, thus being considered a novel medical model that is suitable for the modern society and the development of medicine.

As a matter of course, we cannot deny that new medical models may come into being in future with the further evolution of sciences & technologies and medical technologies and theories; we need to know that the society, the medicine, and medical models are in constant progress.

2. Doctor–patient relationship model

2.1. *Introduction*

Sigerist, a distinguished medical historian, wrote in his book *Henry Sigerist's Medical History* (1959) that "medicine is not so much a natural science as a social one. The purpose of medicine is social. Its purpose is not only to cure diseases and rehabilitate an organism, but also to adapt a person to his surroundings and become a useful member of society. To this end, scientific methods are frequently employed for medicine, but the ultimate goal is still social. Every medical action always involves two types of parties, namely physicians and patients, or more broadly, medical groups and society; medicine is nothing more than a multifaceted relationship between these two groups of people." This statement illustrates the definitions of the doctor–patient relationship in the narrow sense and in the broad sense.

The doctor–patient relationship in the narrow sense refers to the individual relationships between physicians and patients. Starting with patients seeking medical treatment, this relationship enables the medical practice through the information exchange between physicians and patients. In a broad sense, the doctor–patient relationship refers to the relationship between the doctor-centered group of medical personnel and the patient-centered group of patients created during medical treatment. The group of medical personnel comprises physicians, nurses, medical technicians, management personnel and logisticians, while the group of patients consists of patients and their relatives, guardians, employers, and so on.[3] Doctor–patient relationship is a special interpersonal relationship. The definition of interpersonal relationship: First, the direct relationship with us is called interpersonal role relationship; then, the emotional relationship with us is called interpersonal emotional relationship. Humans have to play different roles in different situations and act appropriately under all circumstances.

In essence, physicians and patients are linked into a "communities of interests", because both physicians and patients share the common goal of "conquering disease and getting better as soon as possible"; conquering the disease depends not only on physicians' excellent medical skills, but also on the patients' confidence and active cooperation in conquering the disease. It is the common responsibility of both physicians and patients to fight against diseases. Only when both physicians and patients work closely together and actively cure the diseases, can a favorable therapeutic effect be achieved. Both physicians and patients are in a key position in the process of resisting and curing diseases; the desire of patients to recover should be realized through physicians, who need to intensify their understanding and comprehension of medical science during the diagnosis and treatment of diseases so as to improve their diagnostic and therapeutic skills. In the face of disease, both physicians and patients belong to the "allied forces" and "united front" and have to encourage each other to fight against disease together.

To preserve the harmonious relationship between physicians and patients belonging to the same community of interests, both parties shall

---

[3] Xu, P., Wang, Y., & Cao, Y. (2006). *A study on physician–patient relationship in contemporary China*. Jinan: Shandong University Press.

make concerted efforts. Here is an interesting folklore to illustrate this relationship. There is an ancient story about Sun Simiao, the King of Medicine in the Tang Dynasty. One day, he went out to collect medical herbs in deep mountains, where he encountered a female tiger. His followers thought that the tiger was going to attack them, so they left Sun Simiao and fled. However, Sun Simiao felt that the tiger seemed to be suffering an unspeakable disease. It turned out that the tiger got stuck in her throat by a long bone and was thus extremely uncomfortable, so she tried to see physician Sun Simiao in the road. Soon, Sun Simiao took the foreign body out of the tiger's throat, and the tiger left contentedly. A few days later, when Sun Simiao passed that place again on his way home after the collection of necessary medical herbs, he found that female tiger and her little tigers waiting by the roadside to express thanks. This story illustrates two truths: First, even if a tiger is sick, a physician should treat it in a spirit of benevolence, let alone patients with diseases; hence, physicians should be sympathetic to all patients and actively cure their diseases. Second, since even a man-eating tiger was grateful and responds politely to the physician who relieved her, patients should show fundamental respect and gratitude for the physicians who helped them. In a sense, mutual respect, cooperation, and interdependence are the most fundamental features of physician–patient relationship.

Of course, there are a variety of ways in which physicians interact with patients. In 1956, Szasz and Hollender, both of which were well-known American medical sociologists, proposed three common doctor–patient relationship models, that is, activity–passivity model, guidance–cooperation model, and mutual participation model, by the level of physician's initiative from the perspective of medicopsychology.[4]

2.2. *Four different models*

2.2.1. *Model 1: Activity–passivity model*

In this model, physicians appear as experts with absolute authorities and take the initiative in the relationship between physicians and patients. In

---

[4] Szasz, T. S., & Hollender, M. H. (1976). The physician–patient relationship. In C. Englewood (Ed.), *Moral problems in medicine* (pp. 64–67). NJ: Prentice-Hall Inc.

the meantime, patients are in a passive position, where they completely take orders from physicians. This relationship applies mainly to patients who are not to or are found difficult to express their will such as infants and young children and patients with coma, shock, and severe mental illness. Therefore, such relationship is described as the "relationship between parents and infants". Since patients have no initiative and completely submit to the medical personnel in such a case, the latter shall treat the former with a high sense of responsibility, noble morality, and excellent skills without causing damage to them. Hence, this model is also known as "domination–obedience model".

For instance, when a physician rescues an unnamed patient with coma who is unable to express his/her will and has no family around to help make the decision, the rescue physician should appear as an absolute expert, while the patient has to accept the physician's medical advice and medical actions unconditionally. This is the activity–passivity model of physician–patient relationship. In this model, physicians are allowed to give full play to their technical advantages, while the interests of patients are guaranteed by physicians' conscience. Physicians have to put patients' interests first all the time. If the said physician fails to put the patient's interests first or he is too selfish, adverse consequences may have happened to the patient. Some believe that the "activity–passivity model" involves the lack of respect for patient's autonomy and values; however, from the perspective of modern medicine, this model still has some merits for the patients with poor cognitive or autonomic abilities and no support from relatives or friends or in emergencies.

2.2.2. *Model 2: Guidance–cooperation model*

In this model, both the physicians and the patients have a certain initiative. Although physicians are still authoritative, they only play a guiding role; patients are allowed to ask questions and choose to cooperate with treatment. This relationship applies to the patients who are conscious and able to express their subjective wishes, thus being described as the relationship between "parents and teenagers". Since infants don't have cognitive abilities, they don't resist their parents' decisions; because teenagers have certain cognitive ability, they could choose to cooperate or assist with their parents' directions. This is the difference between "guidance–cooperation model" and "activity–passivity model".

For instance, a patient with stomach cancer turned to a very famous physician in the field; after learning his conditions, the physician gave the patient some guidance based on his own professional experience; upon receipt of the physician's advice, the patient raised his own questions; the physician answered the patient's questions. Although the patient did not fully understand what the physician said, he decided to follow the physician's advice in the end; he accepted to be treated with the physician's program. This is the guidance–cooperation model of physician–patient relationship. In this model, it may still be the physicians who make the difference ultimately, but when compared with the "activity–passivity model", patients participate in decision-making to a certain extent; therefore, the progressive significance of this model is wonderfully remarkable; the interaction between physicians and patients gives full play to the enthusiasm of both sides helps to improve the curative effect, reduce errors and establish a favorable doctor–patient relationship of mutual trust. Of course, the inequality of rights between physicians and patients is still obvious in this model.

2.2.3. *Model 3: Mutual participation model*

In this model, physicians and patients have roughly equal initiative and decision-making power; physicians listen to and respect patients' ideas on an equal basis; physicians and patients work with each other to jointly participate in the decision and implementation of the treatment program. This relationship is applicable to the relationship between physicians and patients with certain medical knowledge or chronic patients who "build up medical knowledge during prolonged illness". For example, against most chronic diseases, physicians tell patients what to do at home, what to pay attention to, what to eat, how to do exercise, and so on; patients will follow physicians' instructions autonomously because chronic patients can't stay in hospitals for a long time. Such relationship is described as one between "adults" and helps to alleviate doctor–patient conflict, break the physician–patient barrier, and establish mutual trust-based doctor–patient relationship.

For instance, a diabetic patient seeks medical advice due to lower limb pain and difficulty in walking. The physician finds that the poor blood glucose control-induced arteriosclerosis obliterans of the lower extremities brought about intermittent claudication. Upon that, the physician suggests several treatment programs based on the patient's conditions, including such means of treatment as surgery, minimally invasive interventional therapy, and physical therapy. After the successful and careful communication with the patient, the two sides agree on a program that they both think was appropriate. This is the "mutual participation model" of physician–patient relationship, and its connotation is actually the participation of both physicians and patients in the selection or decision-making of medical behaviors and the final decision-making. In this model, which represents an ideal physician–patient relationship, both physicians and patients can be satisfied with their moral and responsibility-related requirements. As a matter of course, such a model also needs to be built on a certain basis: Physicians should put their patients' interests first; there should also be effective communication between physicians and patients; physicians should respect the patients' personalities; patients should have full trust in their physicians. The following steps are normally followed for the implementation of "mutual participation model": Physicians inform patients of their medical choices, and that the patients' opinions are important; physicians explain to patients the possible options and the advantages and disadvantages of each option; physicians discuss their preferences with patients and provide support for patients to make consideration; physicians discuss medical preferences with patients, make decisions, and schedule possible follow-ups.

Since the above-noted three doctor–patient models were proposed by American scholars, they can't fully address the medical practice in China. Chinese scholar Cao Kaibin proposed the "consumerism" physician–patient relationship model as a supplement.[5]

2.2.4. *Model 4: Consumerism model*

In this model, patients' initiative is greater than that of physicians; patients give orders to physicians, while the physicians follow such orders. This

---

[5] Cao, K. (1990). *Contemporary medical ethics*. Shanghai: Shanghai People's Publishing House.

relationship is true in some commercial medical institutions such as commercial clinics and pharmacies. The relationship is likened to the relationship between "parents and spoiled child"; parents always give their children what they cry for.

For instance, it's a frequent phenomenon in some retail pharmacies that, when patients buy medicines against their lists, the pharmacists simply dispense the drugs as per such lists; this is a typical "consumerism model", where patients place orders and pay the bill, while medical personnel assist in that process.

Let's look at another typical example. A woman goes to a plastic surgery hospital and requests the physicians to make her eyes look like Zhao Wei's, her nose like Fan Bingbing's, her mouth like Liu Yifei's, and her face like Yang Mi's through plastic surgery. The patient simply wants to be as beautiful as these celebrities, but she knows nothing about the expected effect; however, the plastic surgeons follow her requirements to develop the surgery program without considering whether such plastic surgery in her face is appropriate and beautiful, and without considering the fact that such a complicated operation may lead to a long recovery period; this is also a "consumerism model" of physician–patient relationship. In this model, physicians and patients are like two sides of a commodity trade; patients are fully autonomous, while physicians provide the "commodities" based on patients', or more exactly, customers' requirements. This is not compliant with general medical principles, and the patients without adequate basic medical knowledge are limited in their ability to make medical decisions; this consumerism model is likely to cause hazards ultimately to patients themselves. Take the above-noted woman who asks for plastic surgery as an example; the result is likely to be a beauty who is not what she imagined; however, this is only a minor risk, since she is also likely to experience complications that may even be life-threatening, from extensive plastic surgery.

Medical communication in consulting rooms is accompanied by medical treatment. Since the purposes of the two practices are not the same, not every relationship model exists in such medical communication. Let's have a look at the activity–passivity model first. In this model, patients are infants and young children or cognitively abnormal or in an emergency like a rescue; besides curing diseases and saving lives, there is little room for medical knowledge to spread. Furthermore, patients have the absolute initiative in hands in the consumerism model, while physicians passively cooperate with patients to provide medical services; therefore, active medical communication from physicians is also not practical. Hence, among the above-noted four models of doctor–patient relationship, only the guidance–cooperation model and the mutual participation model are frequently observed in one-to-one medical communication (Table 3.1).

Although patients come from different backgrounds with different levels of education, they often follow a similar learning cycle (Figure 3.2). Seeing a physician is not the end of learning, but the starting point. Patients achieve immediate results through diagnosis and treatment of disease, when anxiety is turned into satisfaction. By sticking to the

Table 3.1   Summary of doctor–patient relationship models.

Type	Physician's position	Patient's position	Scope of application	Similar relationship
Activity–passivity	Absolute authority	Obey the physician completely	Patients have nothing to express or difficult to express the will	Parents and infants
Guidance–cooperation	Physicians still have authorities, but they only play a guiding role	Cooperate with physicians for treatment	Patients who are conscious and able to express subjective wishes	Parents and teenagers
Joint participation	Holding roughly equal initiative and decision-making power	Holding roughly equal initiative and decision-making power	Patients with some medical knowledge	Between adults
Consumerism	Taking orders from patients	Issuing orders	In some commercial medical establishments where patients hold great power	Parents and spoiled children

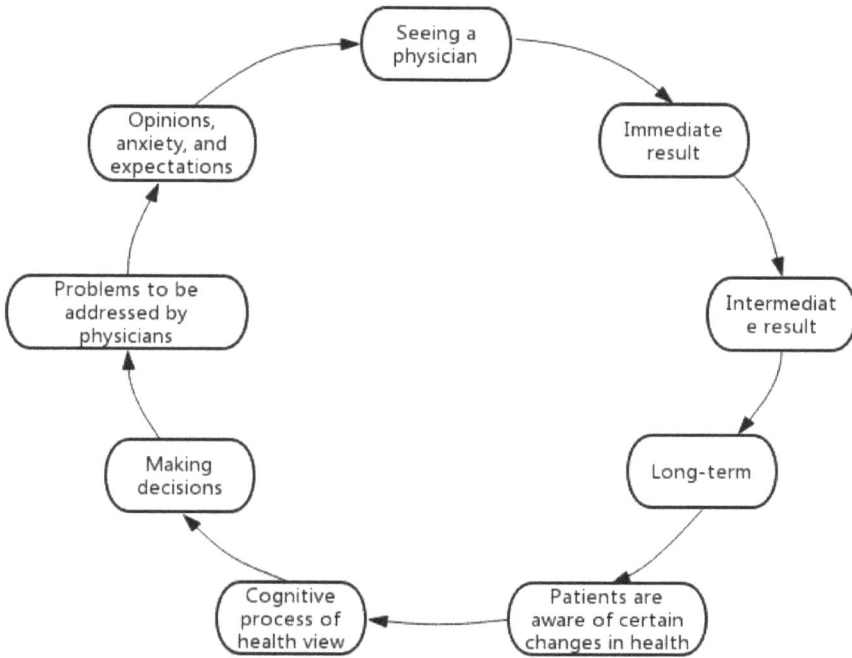

Figure 3.2   Patients' learning cycle (Source: Tate, 2011).

programs, patients get intermediate results; by persevering in doing so, they get long-term results. However, health changes again and the patients become aware. Patients make the decision to take care of themselves or choose health care by learning about health and illness, taking into account the previous experience and consulting families and friends. If there are problems that need to be addressed by physicians, patients will seek medical advice again. This is an iterative process. Therefore, medical communication begins in consulting rooms and can be closely integrated with patients' daily health practices.

3. Process and characteristics of doctor–patient interpersonal communication

Let's take a look at the communication between physicians and patients in consulting rooms. First, the inquisition begins, and the medical personnel

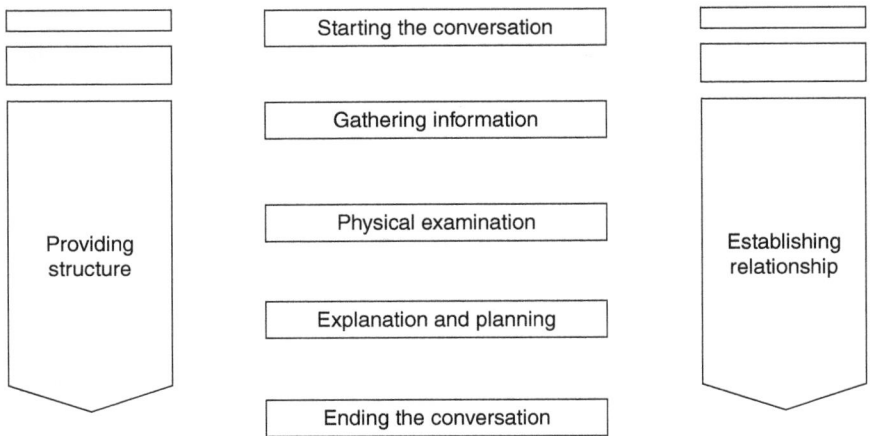

Figure 3.3 Basic framework of Cambridge-Calgary Guide.[6]

begin to gather information. After detailed physical examination, the medical personnel explain and develop a treatment program. The inquisition comes to an end. On the one hand, the physicians shall inform patients of the main content of inquisition; on the other hand, they need to build trust with their patients. This is the Cambridge-Calgary Guide established by scholars Kurtz, Silverman, and Draper (Figure 3.3).

A simple example is presented here. A patient goes to the physician because of dizziness. The talk is initiated. The physician greets the patient and takes his/her name; the physician introduces himself/herself and makes clear the nature and purpose of the interview, gets the patient's consent and shows respect and interest for the patient, checks whether the patient is comfortable and identifies the reason for the patient's visit; the physician needs to gather information about the patient, including the general information about the patient (name, age, nationality, employment status, home address, etc.), and the information about patient's symptoms (chief complaint, history of present illness, past history, family history, disease-related risk factors, etc.), especially the information about the onset and concomitant symptoms of the present dizziness, and the

---

[6] Kurtz, S., Silverman, J., & Draper, J. (Eds.). (2005) *Teaching and learning communication skills in medicine*. Oxford: Radcliffe Publishing.

hypertension and other related risk factors; next, the physician shall perform thorough physical examinations of the patient, especially the physical examinations related to the patient's visit, for example, the physical
examinations of blood pressure and nervous system; the physician needs
to explain the problem and establish a treatment program based on the
obtained information and examination result in order to provide explanation and diagnosis and treatment program associated with patient's view,
find out how the patient thinks and feels about the information given, and
encourage interaction rather than one-way communication; finally, the
talk comes to an end. On the one hand, the physician needs to methodi-
cally set up the complete structure of inquisition during the entire interview or inquisition; on the other hand, he/she needs to establish a
favorable relationship with the patient during the inquisition. This conforms to the basic framework of the Cambridge-Calgary Guide.

Within the basic framework of Cambridge-Calgary Guide, the three
scholars went further to propose the extended framework of the
Cambridge-Calgary Guide (Figure 3.4).[7] Within the extended

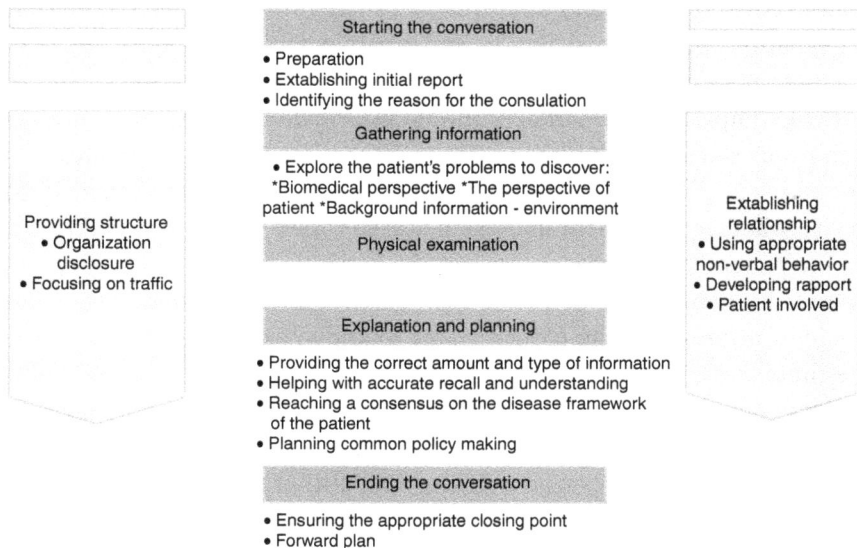

Figure 3.4   Extended framework of Cambridge-Calgary Guide.[7]

---

[7] ibid.

framework, at the beginning of inquisition, the physician needs to get prepared, create the initial report, identify the patient's questions or the questions that the patient wishes to address through appropriate opening questions, listen carefully to the patient's opening statement (do not interrupt the patient or direct the patient's reaction), confirm and identify deeper problems, and negotiate about the agenda for the conversation; this is a time to consider the needs of both the patient and the physician; then, the physician needs to start collecting patient data, explore the patient's problems, encourage the patient to tell stories, use his/her own words to tell the physician how the problem started and developed, use open and closed questioning techniques to appropriately turn questions from open to closed, promote the response of patient by verbal or non-verbal means, clarify if the patient's statement is unclear or needs to be supplemented, and make brief summary; the physician needs to find out specific problems from the biological perspective, the patient's own perspective and the background information, and perform detailed physical examinations, especially related physical examinations; then, the physician needs to explain and plan treatment based on previously collected information; during explanation and treatment planning the physician needs to provide an accurate amount and form of information (give the patient comprehensive and appropriate information; assess the information needs of each individual patient, and create and verify modules: it's necessary to give the patients modular information that they can absorb; verify whether the patient understands, determine how to proceed based on the patient's response, and assess the patient's intention: ask for prior knowledge when giving information to the patient to understand the range of information the patient wants to know; explain at the appropriate time: avoid giving advice, information, or guarantee too early), help patients accurately repeat and understand (plan the illness explanation: break up the explanation into discrete parts, and establish logic sequence; use clear classification or prompts; use repetition and summarization to reinforce information; use concise and easy-to-understand wording: avoid jargon or explanation with jargon; use visual means to convey information), get the patient's understanding (provide explanation and diagnosis & treatment program associated with patient's view, find out how the patient thinks and feels about the information given, and encourage interaction rather than one-way communication), and share treatment program and decision;

All treatment programs require the participation of physician and patient in decision-making (objective: inform the patient of the decision-making process, involve patients in decision-making at the level they want, and enhance the patient commitment to performance of program); explore treatment options, determine the level of participation the patient wishes to have in making the decision, and negotiate to establish a mutually acceptable treatment program; the physician should prepare further planning arrangements at the end of inquisition (make a plan with the patient to contact the physician later; explain possible unintended consequences, the actions to be taken when the program does not work, and when and how to ask for help). The physician needs to, throughout the inquisition, establish a good relationship with the patient by using the behavioral art of using non-verbal communication (e.g. eye contact, facial expressions, and voice cues), and seek development of close relationship (accept the rationality of patients' views and feelings without judgment; communicate, understand and empathize with the patient's feelings or difficulties, and acknowledge the patient's views and feelings clearly and openly; provide support: express concern, understanding, and a desire to help, appreciate patient's efforts to overcome illness and proper self-care, and offer partnerships; handle embarrassing and disturbing topics and physical pain with sensitivity in a considerate manner, including questions related to physical examination); involve the patient in the process (share ideas with and encourage participation of patient); explain the rationale behind the seemingly inconclusive problems or physical examination; explain the process and ask permission during the physical examination, and make sure the consultation is well organized (summarize at the end of each inquiry's specific thread to confirm understanding of the patient's question, and move on to the next link; go from one link to another by using prompts and transitional statements, including laying the groundwork for the next link; organize the interview structure in logical order; pay attention to the schedule and keep the interview on task).

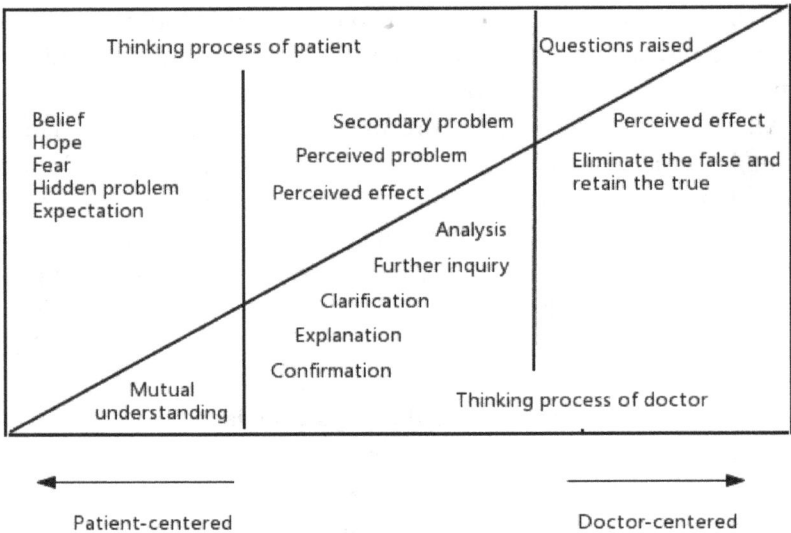

Figure 3.5   Transition model of control over doctor–patient communication style.
Source: Tate, 2011.

Analyzing the thinking processes of medical personnel and patients is one of the ways to learn about the characteristics of doctor–patient interpersonal communication. Peter Tate, a British physician and medical educator, used the following model to conclude the relationship between doctor–patient communication style and thinking process (Figure 3.5).[8] In the doctor-centered doctor–patient communication, doctors are only concerned with the main claims of patients; they eliminate the false and retain the true information during collection of information, gradually clarify the truth of disease, and ultimately validate the disease. As the physician's conversational style gradually moves to the left, the patient's thinking process becomes increasingly acceptable. At the leftmost point, the patient and the physician finally reach a mutual understanding. It is observed from this figure that physicians may be more concerned about biology according to the thinking process of physicians; in addition to biological problems, the patient's thinking process contains many

---

[8] Tate, P. (2011). *The physician's communication handbook* (P. Zhigang & H. Liu, Trans.). Shanghai: Fudan University Press.

psychological and social factors (e.g., beliefs, hopes, fears, expectations, and hidden problems). Thus we note that the bio-psycho-social medical model must be employed in order to really achieve a good understanding between patient and doctor.

Doctor–patient communication is an important step in building a favorable physician–patient relationship. Hippocrates, the Father of Medicine in ancient Greece, said, "physicians have three magic weapons, namely language, medicine, and the scalpel. A physician's words are like his scalpel; they can save lives and hurt people". More than 2,000 years ago, the father of western medicine realized that good physician–patient communication could save patients, while inappropriate physician–patient communication could harm them. The Declaration of Fukuoka issued by the World Federation for Medical Education issued in 1989 also pointed out that "all physicians must learn communication and interpersonal skills, and the lack of resonance (empathy) should be seen as a sign of incompetence, just like the lack of skills. Hence, doctor–patient communication should be considered a required course for physicians". Doctor–patient communication style involves two different models, i.e. "physician-centered" and "patient-centered" models. These two different models reflect different orientations during medical activities, and the patient-centered model is gaining popularity. Physician-centered concept and relationship models were principally from the survey performed by Byrne and Long on over 2,000 patients in the mid-1970s, and its main coverage is as follows: Physicians help patients make decisions; physicians present problems, suggestions, and solutions; physicians point out problems and ask patients to make decisions.[9] In this model, patients' participation is low and physicians' dominance is strong. In the 1980s, McWhinney proposed a patient-centered doctor–patient relationship model that required physicians to view all aspects related to disease and medical treatment from the perspective of patients.[10] Later, Mead and Brower pointed out in their research that

[9] Byrne, P. S., & Long, B. E. (1976). *Doctors talking to patients. A study of the verbal behaviour of general practitioners consulting in their surgeries.* London: HMSO.

[10] McWhinney, I. R. (1981). *An introduction to family medicine.* New York, NY: Oxford University Press.

such patient-centered relationship model is more conducive to the joint exploration of disease symptoms, intensifying the understanding of patients, finding common ground, and improving the physician–patient relationship.[11] In 1983, Berlin and Fowkes proposed the LEARN model of receiving patients, which was also a patient-centered reception model. This model is divided into five steps. First, listen (L); physicians are required to ask open-ended questions, use good questions for guidance, and ask for complete information about the patient's visit, including the information about symptoms, motivation, process, background, and so on. Second, explain (E); physicians are required to follow the "bio-psycho-social medical model" to explain to patients the possible diagnosis and the reasons therefor. Third, acknowledge (A); after the explanation of illness, physicians are required to communicate with patients, allow them to ask questions and raise doubts, and find out if there's a difference in how physicians and patients feel about the illness. Fourth, recommend (R); physicians shall take into account the subjective views and the rationality of medical treatment, and propose specific diagnosis and treatment programs. Fifth, negotiate (N); in the end, patients should be asked if they have any questions about the physicians' recommended diagnosis and treatment programs, and both sides shall perform further consultation in order that the patients fully understand and accept the whole process of diagnosis and treatment. The first, third and fifth steps allow patients to fully express their opinions; the second and fourth steps refer to the patients' opinions for explanation or treatment, and truly embody the centering on patient, thereby realizing favorable communication between physicians and patients.

The medical communication in the consulting room is performed on the basis of diagnosis and treatment of diseases. In the framework of Cambridge-Calgary Guide, the physician–patient conversation moves into the explanation and planning phase after information collection and physical examination. In this phase, physicians provide the correct type and amount of information and help patients accurately recall and understand information; ultimately, they achieve mutual understanding and

---

[11] Mead, N., & Brower, P. (2002). Patient-centered consultations and outcomes in primary care: A review of the literature. *Patient Education and Counseling, 48*, 51–61.

work together to establish patient's disease framework and participate in decision-making. In this process, physicians shall make a reasonable selection of information for targeted medical knowledge popularization based on the medical conditions of patients, which may get twice the result with half the effort.

For instance, a patient comes to the hospital with a dry mouth and significant weight loss. The physician is in the consulting room. First of all, it is necessary to collect complete information about the patient, including the patient's complete medical history, past history, family history, disease risk factors, and so on; then, detailed physical examinations shall be performed. The physician thinks the patient may have developed diabetes based on his medical history and physical examination data obtained. At this point, it's necessary to make an explanation to the patient and develop a treatment program. During the explanation, the physician popularizes the medical knowledge about the prevention and treatment of diabetes based on the patient's conditions. That's one of many examples of medical communication in consulting rooms. As a matter of course, medical communication in the consulting room must be based on favorable communication between physicians and patients. If physicians popularize the corresponding medical knowledge based on patients' conditions and needs while having empathy for them, very good results will be achieved; however, if physicians are completely self-centered and fail to take into account patients' feelings and perform good communication, and provided that they simply instruct the patients about medical knowledge and tell them what needs to be done and what doesn't, there would be a very limited amount of knowledge that patients can ultimately accept.

Good physician–patient communication shall adhere to the following principles: People oriented; principle of good faith; principle of equality; principle of wholeness; principle of confidentiality; principle of feedback; principle of respect; principle of mutual participation. Additionally, attention shall be given to the art of communication; the wording shall create a relaxed atmosphere, and open-ended questions shall be raised; moreover, it's essential to understand problems from the patient's perspective, give the patients timely praise and encouragement, steer the talks, and assure the accuracy of information. In addition to language skills, it's also important to pay attention to the non-verbal skills during doctor–patient communication as follows: Physicians shall dress appropriately, neatly and solemnly; physicians' body position shall be slightly tilted toward the patients at a safe distance; physicians shall look at patients with encouragement and support, and shall nod again and again; physicians' facial expression shall be gentle and kind, and they should smile from time to time; consulting rooms shall be quiet, private and compliant with other required principles.

Chapter 4

Principles and Skills of Doctor–Patient Communication

1. Principles of doctor–patient communication

1.1. *Introduction*

The medical activities carried out in the hospital are mainly disease diagnosis and treatment. At this time, patients are mainly focused on the disease and doctors are deemed more trustworthy. Therefore, if medical communication could be carried out under this occasion, the popularization and promotion of medical knowledge will yield twice the result with half the effort.

Doctor–patient communication refers to the process during which the doctor and the patient exchange medical information and express understanding and requirements for medical activities to meet the health demand of the patient. The medical information contains the patient's disease information that doctors obtained by observing, palpating, percussing, and auscultating for the sake of knowing the disease itself. Medical service information such as medical procedures and expenses is also included for the need of medical service. Information about attitudes toward disease, healthy living concepts, and scientific disease perspectives matters a lot because it decides the way we view the disease. The better communication that patients and doctors have, the stronger the trustworthiness would be. Besides, the relationship between them would be more harmonious.

The US Department of Health and Human Services clearly stated in the *Health People 2010* report that "clear, honest and accurate physician–patient communication with eligible cultural understanding and language expression is the key to medical prevention, diagnosis, treatment, and health management". Therefore, doctor–patient communication was listed as one of the main goals of the report by the US Department of Health and Human Services, which mainly consists of two basic tasks: exchange of information and relationship building. The former should establish in medical treatment, while the latter should focus on patient care.

1.2. *Principles*

Doctor–patient communication usually follows the four basic principles: respect, integrity, empathy, and professionalism.

1.2.1. *Principle of respect*

Respect refers to esteem and value somebody or something. In *The Book of Han — Biography of Xiao Wangzhi*: "Wangzhi was honored as a master. After the emperor took the throne, he banqueted Xiao many times to talk about the governance of the country."

In Jia's *New Account of Political Prose*, Han dynasty: "Relatives and friends of senior officials and nobles, although there is no extraordinary talent, but as long as they respect others, someone will assists them to achieve their goals". Ouyang Xiu, from Song Dynasty, wrote in *The Epitaph of the Huang Cong's Nephew Bo Ping Marquis*: "Respect the teachers and friends, indefatigable in the study of learning".

In the old saying, respect refers to a state of mind and a way of words and deeds that people attach importance to others because others are regarded as higher than their own status, and believes that respecting others is a noble virtue. In modern society, the meaning of respect has gradually been extended to the mentality and words and deeds that treat each other as equal. Respect for others is a good performance of a person's basic qualities, a civilized social method and a cornerstone for carrying out work and establishing good social relationships smoothly. Respect for leaders, colleagues, subordinates, the general public, and other people at all levels is conducive to unity and cooperation and improves working efficiency. Respect for family members is conducive to shaping a harmonious family atmosphere. Respect for friends is conducive to making extensive and lasting friendship. In short, respect for others, life will be more harmonious, more happily.

Therefore, respect is the most basic requirement in the interpersonal contact. The principle of respect is also the most basic principle in the doctor–patient communication. People are equal to each other. Everyone has a need to be respected and to have a sense of self-respect. Regardless of gender, age, high or low in social status, background, what kind of disease they have, or what kind of state they are, they should be respected by medical personnel. Patients should also respect doctors, nurses, and medical technicians. Patients shall not refuse treatment or distrust doctors because of the latter's younger age or lower seniority. Following the principle of respect, medical personnel should respect the patient's wishes and choices too. They shall not look down on the patient with a superior mentality. Especially when the patient raises an objection, they shall not suppress the patient's opinion with an authoritative role.

For example, a patient visits a doctor because of poor glycemic control of diabetes. When the doctor communicates with the patient, he frequently picks up the phone, sends WeChat messages, communicates with other people, does other things, and leaves the patient alone, which is a disrespect for the patient. When the doctor explains the condition, the patient frequently interrupts the doctor's speech, or repeatedly asks the same question, which is disrespect for the doctor.

Similarly, the doctor believes that the patient needs insulin therapy and directly rejects the patient's doubts, telling him that insulin must be taken and there is no other treatment plan and does not take the patient's opinion into consideration, also refuses to understand why the patient does not want to take insulin, which is also disrespect for the patient. The patient doubts the doctor's treatment program and does not communicate with him but questions his professionalism, authority, and medical ethics, which is also disrespect for the doctor.

Mutual respect between people is the primary condition for harmonious coexistence. Without mutual respect from the heart, there will be no good communication; thus it will be difficult for doctors and patients to achieve consistency in the treatment of diseases. Treatment effects can also be affected.

1.2.2. *Principle of integrity*

Integrity indicates to acting faithfully with the thought of sincerity, which contains the meaning of being honest, respecting facts, seeking truth from the facts, and keeping promises. In *The Book of Rites*, Jitong wrote: "A man of virtue offers sacrifices to gods to show his integrity, loyalty, and admiration". From a literal point of view, integrity includes sincerity and faith. Sincerity is mainly referring to the honest moral qualities inside. Faith means credit and trust, which mainly refer to the external manifestation of honesty. Sincerity refers more to the quality of honesty in the heart, and "faith" focuses on the trust for others. The combination of "sincerity" and "faith" forms a vocabulary with both internal and external meanings and rich connotations. Its basic meaning emphasizes honesty and credit, that is, sincerity and faith.

Integrity is a kind of traditional virtue, and a person's essential quality. Integrity is the basic requirement of human beings and the rule of social activities. Physicians and patients should also follow the principle of integrity. Sincerely getting along and mutual trust between physicians and patients are necessary prerequisites for effective communication. Medical personnel should inform their patient about the treatment they offer and its effect faithfully, rather than blindly exaggerate its positive effects, and conceal possible negative effects.

Take responsibility for your commitments and duties. In the same way, patients should not regard treatment as a doctor's business which has nothing to do with themselves, and ignore their own health status. Instead, patients should share the responsibility of restoring health condition with the doctor, tell the true medical history, real thoughts, and the real results after treatment.

For example, one patient was diagnosed with herniation of the lumbar intervertebral disc because of persistent low back pain. Due to the serious symptoms, surgical treatment is required. During the conversation with the patient, it is an exaggeration that if the doctor only told him the benefits of the operation without the possible risks, or told the patient that the operation is absolutely safe and free of any risks. Violation of the principle of integrity in physician–patient communication may lead to deviation in patient decision-making. There is another example, a patient was admitted to the hospital due to a severe infection. During the treatment, various invasive rescue methods such as tracheal intubation and deep vein puncture were performed. However, the patient actually had a history of AIDS for many years. The patient and his family did not tell the doctor. This is also a serious violation of the principle of integrity in doctor–patient communication. In this case, it may cause difficulties in treatment, but also may spread the disease without the medical personnel knowing it. The patient should believe that it is safe to tell the doctor all medical history, because there is also a very important principle of confidentiality in physician–patient communication.

A patient came to the hospital because of chest tightness. After being admitted to the hospital, he was diagnosed with coronary heart disease. Active treatment was performed and his condition was obviously improved. However, the patient told the doctor that his symptoms did not improve because he wanted to stay in the hospital for a few more days. The doctor then re-evaluated his condition and changed other drug treatments. This also violated the principle of integrity in physician–patient communication, which may cause misunderstandings in treatment and unnecessary increase in treatment costs. Sometimes, the violation of the principle of integrity may also threaten the life of the patient. For example, a young girl came to the hospital because of the lower abdominal pain. The doctor asked whether she had a sexual activity and there was a menstrual change. Because the girl is still young, not married, she concealed the history of sexual activity and refused to do gynecological examination. In fact, this girl is suffering from ectopic pregnancy. If she is not treated in time, she will die of hemorrhage.

1.2.3. *Principle of empathy*

Empathy refers to the awareness, grasp, and understanding of other people's emotions, which are mainly related with EQ and embodied in emotional self-control, transposition thinking, listening ability, and expressing respect. Empathy is a psychological concept, which means in order to really understand others, we must take others' perspective to view problems. As the saying goes, to think in others' shoes. "the same heart, the same reason", the Chinese old saying also emphasizes on empathy.

No matter in daily work or life, anyone who has empathy is good at understanding the wishes of others and is willing to understand and help others. Such a person is the most popular and trustworthy of all. The source of conflict between people usually stems from mutual misunder-standings. If both sides can think of the origin of the problem from the perspective of each other, many problems may be solved.

In the current medical environment, patients and doctors have their own difficulties. Therefore, in the medical process, both doctors and patients need to have empathy. On the one hand, it is an indisputable fact that the number of medical personnel is insufficient and the workload is seriously excessed. Hospitals are overloaded, also. On the other hand, patients often complain that the waiting time is too long and the consulta-tion time is too short. In such a medical background, both doctors and patients should follow the principle of empathy and stand on the other side's position.

Doctors should put themselves in the position of patients to treat the disease. Patients should be more considerate of the hard work of medical staff.

As the famous doctor Fei BoXiong from Qing Dynasty said: "If I was sick, what would I want my doctor should do? If my parents, my wife and my children are sick what would I want their doctor should do? When you think about it, the desire for profit becomes weak". It is necessary for doc-tors and patients to think and understand each other so that doctors and patients can communicate effectively.

For example, a patient came to the hospital from a long way. He started queuing early in the morning, waited for hours, and finally got to a specialist number. Then he queued at the door of the clinic for 3 hours and finally got his turn. The expert only gave five minutes of treatment and the patient was dissatisfied. From the patient's point of view, he traveled as far as he can see the expert. Of course, he hopes to tell the experts everything in as much detail as possible, and the expert to diagnose his disease seriously, carefully, and responsibly. In fact, the expert's 5-minute consultation is naturally not enough for the patient. As a doctor, to understand the patient's thoughts, it is necessary to be pleasant and careful when visiting patients, and at the same time, within a limited period of time, to know all the patient's data, give related examinations, make a diagnosis and treatment advice, and tell the patient what to do next. From the point of view of doctors, a half-day expert clinic may have to treat dozens or even hundreds of patients. In order to visit all patients who has already hanged the number, sometimes there is no time to go to the toilet and eat. The five minutes of the consultation were actually squeezed out and saved by the doctor from his spare time. As a patient, it is also necessary to understand the doctor's difficulties. In order to visit all the patients who have been identified, they are all working over-time to visit patients. It is believed that although doctors do not take a long time, doctors will certainly use their professional abilities and advantages to give patients a diagnosis of the disease and further treatment plans during this period. If both parties have empathy and can put themselves in each other's shoes, then the doctor–patient communication will be very smooth and the diagnosis and treatment of the disease is also very beneficial. If both sides only stand on their own perspective, only consider their own difficulties, and do not consider the others' point of view, then there will be obstacles in communication between the two sides and barriers in the diagnosis and treatment of diseases.

1.2.4. *Principle of professionism*

There is a need for professionalism in all professions. Professional spirit means: deep learning and tireless research on work; strive for excellence; constant learning and innovation; full of creativity; beyond the general technical level; enthusiastic pursuit of high client satisfaction.

In medicine, American doctor William Osler believes that the most important trait of doctors can be summarized in the Latin word "Aequanimitas". The meaning of the word includes "kindness" as well as "inner peace", "calm", and "patience". The latter does not mean that doctors are indifferent when they treat the disease. Instead, they are calm and rational through long-term vocational training and, which can bring psychological comfort and security to the patients. And these are professional principles.

Medicine is different from other occupations. Doctors must be benevolent for patients. His "calmness" not only can bring psychological comfort and security to patients, but also let them choose the treatment approach properly and rationally in the process of implementation free from the influence of emotions and the external environment.

In accordance with professional principles, it also includes the principle of confidentiality between doctors and patients. In the process of medical history collection, making a diagnosis and giving treatment, medical personnel have the responsibility to protect the privacy of patients, do not make moral judgments, do not make fun and discriminate against the patient, and respect the patient's self-esteem.

At the same time, the most easily overlooked point is that medical staff should have the ability to immediately separate from the specific medical scene from the professional point of view, maintain their own rational and mental health, and do not cause their own psychological harm due to exposure to childbirth, old age, illness, and injury.

Professionalism is required in any profession, as is the doctor. For example, when a doctor receives a patient with a terminal tumor, the general situation is very poor and there is no indication of surgery at all. However, the patient's family members still require surgical treatment. At this time, the doctor should analyze the patient's specific situation in detail to the patient's family members with his own professional spirit and inform them the advantages and disadvantages of the operation and the reasons for the current non-surgical. On the other hand, the doctor should comfort the family members, choose the most appropriate treatment for the patient at present, rather than blindly surgery. If the patient dies after treatment, the doctor should not fall into bad emotions. Instead, he should view the patient's death scientifically and continue to treat the next patient.

The content of professional principles covers a lot. There are also professional rules to be followed in Western country health systems. For example, medical staff cannot use their medical resources to seek convenience for their relatives, because most patients do not have such facilities and they must follow the procedure. If medical staff use the advantages of working in medical institution to arrange their relatives jumping the queues, it is a violation of the principle of medical fairness and it is unfair to other patients. For another example, medical staff cannot treat their relatives. This does not simply mean that relatives cannot be facilitated, but that in the treatment of their relatives, especially close family members, the emotion and judgment of medical staff may be affected by external factors and become no longer objective and the "calm" and "coolness" under normal circumstances are lost, which is extremely unfavorable for patient treatment. Medical staff and patients cannot have intimate relationships beyond friendship. If medical staff use their profession to request an improper intimate relationship with patients, they will be notified or even disqualified.

1.2.5. *Other principles*

In addition to the above four core principles, doctor–patient communication should also abide by the following principles:

1.2.5.1. People-oriented

The development of modern society takes people as the core and meets people's needs as the value orientation. The new development theory centered on the unified and harmonious development of man and nature has aroused widespread concern in society. When people seek medical treatment, they not only need to get timely and effective treatment in physiology, but also need to receive psychological attention, respect, and understanding. The modern medical model has changed from a purely biomedical model to a bio-psycho-social medical model. In this model, the patient-centered and the principle of people first are well suited to the contemporary medical model. In the doctor–patient communication, we should start from patient's needs and give them enough humanistic care and finally achieve the patient-centered communication. For example, a patient has a stomach ulcer and visits a doctor. After detailed medical history, the doctor learned that the patient's stomach ulcer is not only related to his eating habits, for instance, ignoring dinner and preferring spicy food, but also related to the pressure of work and the long-term stress in the mental state. In addition to adjust unhealthy habits in the diet, it is also necessary to psychologically give patients some mental adjustment and suggest appropriate slowdown of the work rhythm. Only by comprehensively considering the patient's condition from the physiological-psychological-social perspective and taking the patient as the center, the humanistic care in doctor–patient communication could be reflected, which also is positive for the treatment of the patient. Another example is an elderly female patient who has recently been conscious of chest tightness. She came to the hospital for related examinations and was basically ruled out the patient's organic heart disease. However, the patient still has persistent chest tightness. At this time, the doctor should pay attention to the problems that are not found, instead simply classify the patient as making a fuss about an imaginary illness.

After the doctor's careful excavation, he found that the patient's daughter is in her 30s and has been busy with her career and not married. The situation of her daughter has become the patient's mental anguish. Recently, the daughter of the patient's good friend had married and had children, which touched the patient's worry and caused her chest tightness. At this time, the doctor should relieve the patient's emotions and solve her psychological problems. Naturally, it solved her symptoms. Such medical behavior truly embodies the principle of putting people first.

1.2.5.2. The principle of equality: Both doctors and patients are equal

The patient is first a man in society, then a patient who needs help, and the doctor is also a man in society first, and then a person who can give help to the patient. The traditional doctor–patient relationship is dominated by doctors. For patients, doctors appear as absolute authority, giving patients little chance to speak, which may affect the communication effect between the two parties. As the communication process between people, equality is the first principle, and so in doctor–patient communication.

In doctor–patient communication, whether it is a doctor or a patient, they are all people in society but play different roles. Both sides need to be understood and respected. Therefore, good communication between the two parties must be established on the basis of equality.

At the same time, the principle of equality is also reflected in the fact that regardless of the status and rank of the patient, they should be treated equally.

For instance, when a senior official and an civilian come to an expert at the same time, the number of civilian ranks in front of the official, so the civilian should be seen first, instead of letting the official cut the queue. At the same time, for both the civilian and officials, the distribution of doctor's time and the choice of doctor's order should be based on the severity and complexity of the disease, not on the level of the status. Official should not be placed in front of civilian or take longer treatment time because of their status.

If there were two patients in the emergency room at the same time, one was a senior official, but his condition was relatively stable, the other was a civilian and his condition was very serious. At that time, there was only one doctor in the emergency room. The doctor should first rescue and treat the critically ill civilian, rather than the official. Seemingly, during the process of medical treatment, both doctors and patients are equal in their relations. As doctors, they cannot be servile or agree patient's unreasonable requirements because the other party is an official. Doctors cannot look down on the other side, make a superior posture, ignore the reasonable demands of patients, because the other party is a civilian. As a doctor, regardless of the identity and status of the other party, he should treat the patient's illness from his own professional point of view, give appropriate and objective treatment advice and treatment implementation without judging the patient's personal data and background.

1.2.5.3. The principle of wholeness

Human beings are different from machines and cannot be regarded as a simple combination of organs. In the treatment of a body organ, other adjacent and related organs need to be considered. At the same time, with the development of society, people's psychological pressure is constantly increasing and social roles are constantly changing. There are many diseases that not only are biological but also involve psychological and social factors. Therefore, in doctor–patient communication, it is necessary to treat patients as a whole composition. Not only to take natural attributes of patients into account, but also to consider the social attributes of patients, and to communicate from aspects of biology, psychology, and society and to provide integrated and comprehensive medical services.

The patient is not a machine, which cannot be treated simply by splitting it into specific organs. For example, a patient suffering from cerebral infarction, that is, stroke hemiplegia, has to stay in bed for a long time. If we follow the principle of the machine, we just need to treat the brain. In fact, because of a stroke, the swallowing function is impaired so the patient may have a food aspiration and a lung infection. It may also cause skin infections and bedsores due to long-term bed rest. Therefore, when treating the patient, all possible problems need to be taken into account. The holistic treatment, in the treatment of cerebral infarction, must also prevent and control the emergence of pneumonia and bedsores. Meanwhile, because the patient suffered from hemiplegia after a stroke, he not only lost the ability of work but also lost the ability of living independently. He had to rely on other's care. During the patient's treatment and rehabilitation, doctors need to provide psychological counseling to help the patient adapt to the current state and avoid depression after a stroke. On the other hand, it is also necessary to teach his family members who take care of him about routine post-stroke care knowledge to help patients and their families to smoothly pass through the development stage of the disease, try to avoid various post-stroke complications, and strive to help patients get functional partial recovery.

1.2.5.4. Principle of confidentiality

The most significant principle in physician–patient communication which is often overlooked is confidentiality. In physician–patient communication especially when the doctors collect patient's medical history, sometimes it involves lots of patient's privacy that the patient does not want to be known by others. Out of trust for the doctor, the patient informs the private matter to the doctor, and the doctor should keep this confidential because of respect for patient. Doctors should not reveal the patients' privacy or ridicule or discriminate against patients. If the principle of confidentiality cannot be achieved in doctor–patient communication, it will damage the patient's self-esteem; on the other hand, it will endanger the doctor's reputation.

For example, an AIDS patient told his medical history to his doctor. If the doctor reveals the medical history to other patients nearby, this may cause panic among other patients, and also cause other patients to despise and scold the patient. It is a serious violation of the principle of confidentiality in doctor–patient communication. In this case, if the doctor wants to protect other patients, it is entirely possible to transfer the AIDS patient to a single ward or a ward with special protective measures in a low-key and safe way, rather than publicizing the patient's condition.

Another example is a patient who has a terminal tumor and has few days last. During the treatment process, the patient asked not to inform his relatives, including his wife and children and other immediate family members. Then, the medical staff should comply with the principle of confidentiality for the patient. Without the patient's permission, the doctor cannot reveal the patient's condition to anyone, even the closest person.

The principle of confidentiality also includes the understanding that doctors cannot freely reveal information about patients and their conditions, and cannot use the information for profit. For example, after a woman gave birth in a hospital, medical staff disclosed her information to a milk powder manufacturer, causing the milk powder manufacturer to send a large number of advertisements to the woman. This is not only a violation of the principle of confidentiality, but also a violation of national laws and is suspected of trafficking in personal information. Sometimes, the condition of some patients is very complex and has considerable research value. If the doctor needs to use the patient as a research object, he must obtain the written consent of the patient or the agent of the patient. In the meantime, doctors should ensure that all kinds of information of the patient are kept secret during the research process, and the basic information of the patient, such as the name, workplace, should not be disclosed when the research results are published.

1.2.5.5. The principle of feedback

Feedback refers to the speaker passing information to the listener through the language, and the listener passing the information back to the speaker in some way, so that the speaker's intention is confirmed or changed. Without a good feedback mechanism, two sides of communication may have completely different understandings of the same issue. The doctor–patient communication is a two-way communication process, and due to the complexity and profound medical knowledge, most people are lacking basic medical common sense and medical knowledge. In the process of communication, doctors need to use positive feedback to understand whether patients fully understand the doctor's intention or misunderstand it. If there is no feedback, it is very possible that not only the patient completely misunderstood the doctor's original intention, but also the doctor did not know it. There is a great influence on the next treatment.

For example, a patient with diabetes visits a doctor and is told that he needs dietary control, but the patient does not know how to achieve the goal of controlling blood sugar through dietary control. The patient thinks that as long as he does not eat sweets, he gets dietary control. Therefore, the doctor should inform the patient in a concise manner in the process of doctor–patient communication, and at the same time get feedback to know how much the patient understands what the doctor has told him, so as to help the patient's blood sugar management. As a simple example, a diabetic patient was overweight and lacked exercise. The doctor told him that he needed diet control, less carbohydrates, daily calorie intake control, and more exercise. So, the patient begins to eat only one meal a day. Within a few days, the patient became dizzy with hunger, unable to go to work and even fainted with hypoglycemia. The patient apparently did not grasp the essentials of dietary control. Therefore, the doctor should teach the patient how to control his diet and listen to feedback to know how much the patient really knows about diet control. This will ensure that the patient can be correct and effective in his own diet management. Otherwise, not only will it not have a positive effect, but it may also lead to adverse side effects.

Another example is that a patient was found to have lymphoma during the examination. The doctor told him that he had non-Hodgkin's lymphoma. The patient thought that "tumor" was not "cancer" and thought it was a benign disease. He did not pay attention to it, nor did he take active treatment and follow-up, and therefore missed the best time for treatment. In fact, non-Hodgkin's lymphoma is a very common malignant tumor of the blood system. The incidence of malignant tumors in China ranks in the top ten. This is a typical example of a doctor who fails to listen to patients' feedback when telling them of the illness, leading to delays in the treatment of patients.

1.2.5.6. The principle of co-participation

Medical decision-making is often very difficult and important. In the whole process of diagnosis and treatment of patients, both doctors and patients need to participate in the entire process and communicate well. Medical staff should listen to patients' opinions patiently, let patients participate in decision-making together, make judgments and explanations by asking various situations, and inform patients of further diagnosis and treatment plans. Patients can communicate and discuss with doctors when they have different opinions from the plan. When listening to the patient's ideas, it is also necessary to maintain good communication with the patient's family, to inform them of the patient's diagnosis and treatment plan, so that the family can also fully understand the patient's specific situation and participate in discussions and decisions.

For example, a patient with acute cholecystitis needs surgery. There are two options for surgery. One is minimally invasive surgery, and the other is conventional transabdominal surgery. Each has its own advantages and disadvantages. The doctor should tell the patient in detail about both options and discuss with the patient. In the end, it is decided that a more favorable surgical plan is considered by both parties. This is the embodiment of the principle of joint participation. Compared with the absolute authority of the medical side, the joint participation of both doctors and patients has a good effect on the construction of a good physician–patient relationship.

Another example is that an elderly patient has diabetes, and the use of oral hypoglycemic drugs is very unsatisfied. The doctor judges that insulin needs to be injected according to the condition. But in the process of communicating, the doctor finds that the patient is too old to inject insulin on his own, and the patient's families do not live with the patient and cannot inject insulin daily for him. Doctors need to discuss with the patient and his family, then choose a treatment plan that is beneficial to the patient and can be accepted by the patient and his family. By this time, the advantages of joint participation and joint decision-making are reflected.

2. Skills of doctor–patient communication

The skills to communicate with patients have always been regarded as an indispensable skill for doctors. Hippocrates regards the importance of communication as equal to that of medicine and surgery, and calls them the three magic weapons of doctors. In March 1989, *Fukuoka Declaration*, the World Federation of Medical Education pointed out: "all doctors must learn to the skill of communicating and dealing with interpersonal relationship. Lack of resonance should be seen as the same as lack of technology, which is not capable of performance". Medical communication must be based on good physician–patient communication. Words are not only the most important magic weapon for medical staff, but also a double-edged sword. There is an old Chinese saying: warm words make people feel warm even in the cold winter. Harsh words make people feel cold even in summer. Words are not honey, but sweeter than honey; not poison, but worse than poison; not flowers, but more beautiful than flowers; not swords, but sharper than swords. Knife wounds heal in a week, but words hurt, maybe never heal. A word of encouragement from the doctors can turn the patient's worries into happiness, multiply his spirit, and immediately improve his condition. On the contrary, a discouraged speech can also make a patient feel depressed, anxious, bedridden, or even die.

In the process of interpersonal communication, there are two kinds of information: one is verbal information, and the other is non-verbal information. Communication experts point out that less than half of human communication is accomplished through speech, and more than half of information is transmitted through non-verbal means such as intonation, expression, body movements, and so on. Therefore, in the process of face-to-face communication between doctors and patients, both kinds of information need equal attention.

2.1. *Verbal communication*

When collecting disease information, patients and doctors often have incomprehensible situations because of different discourse systems. Therefore, Levenstein (1989) and Steward (2003) put forward the disease-illness model in order to consider both doctors and patients (Figure 4.1).

Patient ask questions
↓
Gathering information
↓
Seek the following two frameworks at the same time

Interweave the two frameworks

Disease framework (Biomedical Perspective)		Patient framework (Patients' Perspective)
Symptom Sign Examination Pathological results		Idea Worry Expectaion Emotions and Thoughts The impact on life
differential diagnosis	Integrating two frameworks ↓	Understanding the patient's illness experience

Explanation and Planning
Understanding and Participating in Decision Making Together

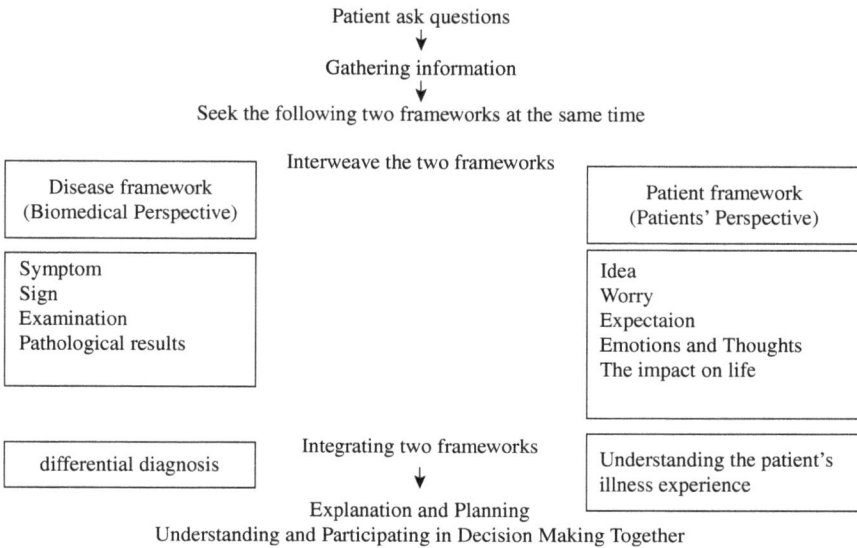

Figure 4.1   Disease-illness model.

Silverman J, Kurtz S, & Draper J. (2009). *Physician–patient communication skills* (X. Yang, Trans.). Beijing: Chemical Industry Press.

"Disease" is the discourse system of doctors, aiming at explaining the biomedical causes of "illness" in terms of pathophysiology. "Illness" is the unique disorder experience of the patient, including his own feelings, thoughts, worries, expectations, emotions and thoughts, the impact on life, and so on. The same disease, different people maybe have different "illness" experiences. The doctor's duty is to find out the symptoms, to treat the disease, and to take care of the patient's "illness" experience. Such communication requires doctors to use both rational and perceptual word to complete it. In order to achieve proper doctor–patient communication, medical ethics requires that doctors should be good at using five languages: polite, explanatory, comfortable, encouraging, protective, and body language. Some scholars believe that the special language requirements in clinical medicine include being good at listening, avoiding stimulation, encouraging appropriately, asking questions correctly, observing carefully, and learning to smile. They also point out that the above requirements should "cohere the harmony and unity of truth, goodness and beauty".

When communicating with patients, doctors should pay attention to the following points:

(1) Create a relaxed atmosphere:
When patients seek help from doctors, they may feel nervous because of unknown illness and lack of medical knowledge, as well as being in unfamiliar surroundings with strange people. Doctors should use gentle gestures and friendly words to relieve the patient's nerves, so that they can confidently tell the doctor the basic information. In addition, when talking with patients, doctors should also pay attention to the necessary etiquette, and should not frequently answer the phone or be disturbed by other things. On the one hand, it is disrespectful to patients. On the other hand, it may aggravate patients' uneasiness. If doctors need to answer the necessary telephone, they should inform patients with appropriate words and obtain their understanding.

(2) Listen to patients initiatively:
When a patient talks to a doctor, the doctor should give the patient a certain degree of autonomy, so that the patient can fully express his opinions. Listen carefully, patiently and attentively to the content and process of the patient's statement. Make patients feel safe and trust doctors. Doctors should also listen carefully to all the ideas expressed by patients, give patients full respect when listening, not to interrupt the expression of patients and judge patients' statements casually. The painful emotions caused by illness should be understood, sympathized, and cared in order to enhance patients' interest and initiative in conversation.

(3) Guide the direction of conversation:
In doctor–patient communication, doctor is in the domination. Doctors not only should listen to patients but also should be good at guiding the direction of the conversation. Doctor should use directive word skillfully and appropriately to guide patient to clearly narrate the evolution of their medical history and the changes of their condition, to make the process of the communication smooth and to obtain the information successfully. When patient complains a lot of irrelevant issues, doctor should change the subject properly, avoid wasting both sides' time, and make the communication more efficient.

(4) The accuracy of information:

When communicating with patients, important information must be confirmed. On the one hand, doctors must be accurate about the details they tell patients, whether in diagnosis or treatment, and cannot provide the wrong information. When the diagnosis and treatment plan is uncertain, as a doctor, should tell the patient that the current state is not clear, should not be specious, and should not make mistakes on important issues. On the other hand, the doctor also needs to confirm the information that the patient told, for the wrong information may mislead the doctor's treatment plan, leading to adverse outcomes.

(5) Use plain language:

Doctors are professionally trained personnel, often using medical terms, but patients are generally lacking of medical knowledge. If doctors only use medical terms to communicate with patients, this may be difficult to understand, and may even cause misunderstanding. Therefore, in doctor–patient communication, doctors should pay attention to the use of easy-to-understand words, coupled with image metaphor, so that patients can easily understand. For example, if a patient is suffering from stroke, the doctor tells his family that the patient had a stroke, the family may not fully understand it. If the doctor tells the patient's family that the patient's blood vessel of the brain is blocked, it will be easier for the patient's family to understand.

2.2. *Non-verbal communication*

Medical staff should recognize relevant clues from patients' non-verbal information, and also realize that their non-verbal information will affect the success of the inquiry and the effectiveness of medical communication. The clues of non-verbal communication include the points below.

Posture: sitting, standing, straightening, relaxing. Body posture can often convey the information of individual emotional state and reflect the attitudes and desires of both sides of the conversation. As a doctor, when communicating with patients, he should relax in sitting posture, lean forward slightly, and nod frequently to make the patient feel that the doctor is friendly and is willing to listen to his illness situation.

Space: use of space, including physical distance and location with communicators. In physician–patient communication, doctors should avoid getting too close or looking directly at patients, which will cause patients' urgency and tension, and should not be too alienated, which will make patients feel that doctors do not care enough. The appropriate space should be for both doctors and patients to maintain a certain distance, so that the eyes can freely contact or separate.

Touch: handshake, pat, physical contact during physical examination. When the patient is tense or agitated, the doctor can pat the patient on the shoulder or shake hands appropriately to ease the patient's mood. However, doctors should avoid inappropriate touching to patients, especially patients of the opposite sex, in order to avoid misunderstanding or harassment.

Action: hand and arm posture, fidget, nodding, foot and leg movements. When the patient tells the state of the illness, the doctor can nod slightly to encourage the patient to continue. If the doctor is restless or answers the phone frequently, the patient will think the doctor does not respect him.

Facial expression: raising eyebrows, frowning, smiling, crying. When the patient tells his painful experience, the doctor's facial expression should be solemn to show his understanding and sympathy. When the patient tells his happy experience, the doctor shall also smile to show that he understands the patients' happiness. A doctor who always smiles makes patients feel friendly and more willing to communicate with him.

Eye action: eye contact, gaze, stare. When communicating with patients, eyes should show honesty and care for patients. It's polite to look at each other when you talk, but long-time direct vision can also cause stress and urgency to the other person and make the patient uncomfortable.

Voice: speed, volume, rhythm, silence, pause, and intonation. When communicating with patients, the voice of doctors should be gentle and firm, and avoid making the patient feel uncertain.

Time: early, late, on time, overtime, slow response, and rapid response. When communicating with patients, doctors should follow the time of appointment. Punctuality is a good reflection of doctors' professionalism.

And in communication, too short and hasty time should also be avoided, which will make patients feel that doctors don't pay attention to them.

Appearance: race, sex, body shape, clothing, dress, temperament. Patient's first impression of the doctor comes from the doctor's clothes and overall image. If a doctor dresses sloppily, it will make the patient feel that the doctor can't be trusted. When an obese doctor requires patients to control their diet, increase their exercise and improve their lifestyle, patients are bound to question the professionalism of doctors, because doctors themselves do not manage their own body shape well. Therefore, as a professional doctor, we should dress appropriately, neatly, and generously and pay attention to the management of body shape.

Environment: location, furniture layout, light, temperature, color. The occasion of physician–patient communication should be quiet, with a certain degree of privacy, to avoid the involvement of unrelated personnel.

2.3. *Differences between verbal and non-verbal communication*

Two communication scientists have summed up several differences between verbal and non-verbal communication.

First of all, the starting point and ending point of word communication are usually very clear, and we know when information processing will finish. Verbal communication is discrete and can be divided into different stages. However, non-verbal communication is continuous, as long as both sides are present, it will continue. Non-verbal communication continues even when there is no verbal communication. Paul Watslavik, a professor at Stanford University, has said: People cannot stop communicating.

Secondly, the mode of verbal communication is relatively single, either through auditory (conversation) or visual (writing). Non-verbal communication can carry on simultaneously through multiple modes, and all our senses can participate in receiving non-verbal information. For example, we can smell each other's scent at the same time, see each other's facial expression, hear each other's voice and intonation, and touch each other's skin and so on.

Thirdly, verbal communication can be actively controlled with clear purpose. However, a lot of non-verbal information is emitted by our unconsciousness. So it is more likely to "leak" the spontaneous clues that we do not realize. These non-verbal messages better reflect our true feelings than the word we have thought over. For example, although the words are compliment, but the face may have inadvertently made a disdainful expression.

Finally, verbal information is more effective for communicating our rational ideas and opinions; yet, non-verbal information is responsible for communicating attitudes, emotions, and feelings. Therefore, in many situations where emotional ties need to be established, non-verbal information plays an important role.

2.4. *Two major tasks of doctor–patient communication*

Medical communication can be carried out in face-to-face doctor–patient communication on the basis of the two major tasks of information collection and relationship establishment in a limited time.

Firstly, information collection is accomplished by exploring patients' problems. The general steps are as follows:

Narration: Doctors should encourage patients to narrate their stories in their own words, from the initial occurrence to the current situation, to find out the reason for this visit.

Questioning: The doctor needs to use appropriate questioning techniques and use open and closed questions, especially question the patients from open questions to closed questions gradually.

Listening: The doctor shall listen carefully and try not to interrupt the patient's statement, and give the patient enough time to think, or pause before continuing.

Response: Respond verbally or non-verbally to the patient's narrative, such as encouragement, silence, repetition, overview and interpretation, etc.

Clues: Receive verbal and non-verbal cues from patients, such as body word, facial expressions, voice cues, and verify these cues, and approve them at the appropriate time.

Exploration: In order to fully understand the patient's point of view, the doctor should actively and appropriately explore the patient's thoughts, the patient's worries about a problem, the patient's expectations or goals, and the impact of each problem on the patient's life.

Encouragement: Encourage patients to express their feelings.

Clarification: Check the vague information and let the patient supply the detailed information. For example, How do you feel when you have a headache?

Confirmation: Confirm the date and sequence of events. Confirm that the information provided by the patient is accurate.

Summary: Periodically summarize to confirm the understanding of the patient's statement and ask the patient to make corrections to the explanation and provide further information.

During this period, doctors should try to use concise and understandable questions and comments, and if using terminology, the terminology should be fully explained. Use abbreviations as little as possible and use full names. The confusing concepts of patients should be summarized and shared with colleagues in time. For example, in gynecological examination, patients often do not understand the difference between "menstrual period" and "between menstruation". Doctors should not take it for granted that patients know the meaning of the term and need to explain it if necessary.

2.5. *Now let's learn the skill for building physician–patient relationship*

2.5.1. *Skills 1: Establish a harmonious atmosphere*

Acceptance: Accept the rationality of the patient's opinions and feelings, without evaluation.

Empathy: To understand and support patients' feelings or situations, and to publicly approve patients' views and feelings. In the current medical environment, patients are likely to accumulate resentment, which may occur before entering the clinic, such as due to unfamiliar procedures. Doctors should understand the patient's anger.

Support: Express care, understanding, and willingness to help patients, and recognize the efforts of patients.

Sensitivity: Carefully handle embarrassing or annoying topics and physical pain, including physical examination-related issues.

2.5.2. *Skills 2: Patient participation*

Share ideas: Share ideas with patients and encourage their participation. For example, "What I'm thinking about right now is..."

Explain the basic principles: Explain the basic principles of problems or physical examination, so as not to appear subjective.

Physical examination: In the process of physical examination, the process should be explained and ask for patient's permission.

2.5.3. *Skills 3: Communication with appropriate non-verbal skills*

Demonstrate appropriate non-verbal behavior, including sightseeing, facial expression, posture, position, action, voice cues, such as speed, volume, intonation, etc.

Use of Notes: If you want to read, write or use a computer, be careful not to interfere with the conversation.

Extraction of patients' non-verbal cues: To obtain information from patients' non-verbal cues, including body language, voice, facial expression, doctors should verify and recognize in good time.

3. Skills of nurse–patient communication

The medical communication in the clinic not only depends on doctors, but also requires the active participation of nurses.

As the saying goes, "thirty percent treatment, seventy percent nursing". Among the medical staff, nurses have the longest contacting time with patients, and the relationship of them is also the closest. If we can effectively carry on medical communication by nurses, we might yield twice the result with half the effort.

What is the nurse–patient relationship and communication?

3.1. *Nurse–patient relationship and communication*

The nurse–patient relationship is the relationship between nurses and patients in the process of medical care practice. It is characterized by workability, professionalism, and helpfulness. In a narrow sense, the nurse–patient relationship is the relationship between nurses and patients. In a broad sense, the nurse–patient relationship also includes the relationship between the nurse and the patient's relatives, escorts, guardians, organizational units, and so on. Modern nursing has evolved from the simple implementation of medical care in the past to the level of comprehensive holistic care including physical, psychological, and social relationships. Therefore, the nurse–patient relationship includes not only technical relationships but also non-technical relationships.

The technical relationship is the helping behavior relationship established by nurses in providing professional nursing activities for patients. This is the basis of the nurse–patient relationship.

The non-technical relations are the multiple relationships including morality, interests, law, culture, and values and so on, formed on the basis of technology, mainly reflected in medical ethics and service attitudes.

The nurse–patient relationship firstly is a working relationship: Establishing a good nurse–patient relationship is a requirement of nursing staff occupation. The interaction between nurses and patients is a professional behavior, which is mandatory, and nursing staff should strive to establish good relationships with patients.

The nurse–patient relationship is also a kind of trust relationship: The nurses and patients need mutual respect and place oneself in others' position and mutual trust. Because of the trust, the patients tell the nurses without reservation about their illness in order to treat the disease. Similarly, nurse also needs to respect and trust patients, and wholeheartedly serve patients from the point of humanistic care.

The nurse–patient relationship is also a therapeutic relationship. Many treatment decisions made by doctors require nurses to participate in the implementation, such as infusion, issuing medicine, etc. Many investigations have shown that good nurse–patient relationship can effectively alleviate or eliminate the pressure from the environment, and the treatment process and the disease itself, help to cure and accelerate the recovery process of the disease. Of course, the nurse–patient relationship is a special, therapeutic relationship that should be carefully implemented, because the therapeutic relationship is focusing on the needs of the patient. In addition to the general life experience factors, the quality, professional knowledge, and skills of nurses will also affect the development of therapeutic relationships. Therefore, it is not only necessary to improve the professional and technical skills of nursing personnel (for example, the ability to get the right idea), but also to learn and advocate the spirit and concept of "Humanized care".

Finally, the nurse–patient relationship is a contractual relationship. Both the nurse and the patient are independent individuals with their own rights and interests. They are premised on respecting each other's rights and fulfilling their respective obligations. They are faithful to each other's commitments in a contractual manner within the framework of the law.

The purpose of nurse–patient communication, firstly, is to establish a well-maintained nurse–patient relationship, so that patients can reduce the loneliness of being alienated and trapped.

Secondly, it is to help patients to correctly understand their own health condition, adjust themselves in a difficult situation, improve their self-control ability, and reduce their dependence on others. Thirdly, it is to collect patient data for a health assessment to determine the patient's health problems.

Finally, it can share information, thoughts, and emotions, and implement care activities for the health problems of patients.

Compared with time-limited doctor–patient communication, the nurse–patient communication is more important in terms of patient care because it has more communication opportunities. At the same time, many patients are more likely to communicate with nurses because the latter are mostly women and have natural and amiable attributes.

However, comparing with doctors, nurses may be less authoritative in the minds of patients, so it may also bring various challenges to nurses in communication.

Therefore, in addition to the principles of nurse–patient communication mentioned in the previous section, there are also the following aspects to be noted:

(1) Conversation

During the conversation, the nurse needs to be both polite and professional. Enhance the popularity of the professional language, using medical terms as little as possible; if you have to use it, you need to make enough explanations. For example, when a nurse prepares to give a patient intravenous or intramuscular injection, she should say that it is a normal injection for the patient to understand. When a nurse gives the patient intravenous rehydration, if the patient is informed of the need for intravenous rehydration, the patient may have difficulty understanding, but if it is to have transfusion, the patient can understand it well. At the same time, when communicating with patients, nurses must use simple, clear-cut statements to express their meaning. Do not use ambiguous words to let patients guess. For example, when a nurse tells the patient that aspirin needs to be taken in the morning, the patient will have doubts about whether it is before or after breakfast. At this time, the nurse should clearly tell the patient that aspirin needs to be taken half an hour before breakfast. The information received by the patient is clear. There would be no misunderstanding or doubt.

In addition, when talking with patients, nurses should also pay attention to the sense of proportion. Nurses have to aware what should be said, what should not be said and to what extent, and they need to be consistent with the doctor. For instance, there is an elderly patient with advanced tumors, but the patient does not know the condition, and the family members of the patient also ask the doctor not to let the patient know for the time being. If the nurse talks to the patient during clinical care, telling the patient that he has advanced cancer, not only violates the principle of sense of proportion, but also violates the principle of confidentiality of the patient's condition, and may also hit the patient's mental state. It is very unfavorable for the patient's treatment.

(2) Listening

Although nurses are less authoritative in the eyes of patients, they feel more intimate. Some situations that patients do not want to share with the doctors, may be willing to tell the nurses. Therefore, the nurse should also pay attention to listening to the patient's thought. In face-to-face communication, listening is as important as the conversation itself. Listening patiently, encouraging patients to fully express information and emotions, which can help build trust between nurses and patients.

Listening is not only about the language itself, but also through the expressions, intonation and other non-verbal information, to understand the patient's true feelings and ideas. The skills include:

- Maintain eye contact and communicate to express your interest in the other's words.
- Maintain a proper position and body distance to avoid distracting movements.
- Use verbal and non-verbal information to encourage patients to state health appeal, express respect for patients, enhance patient self-esteem and their sense of self-worth.
- Do not casually interrupt the patient's statement.
- Guide the patient's statements. If the patient overstates the content that is not related to the condition and treatment, the nurse can appropriately guide the patient's subject to what the nurse needs to know, and control the overall time, so that the patient can fully express his true will. Do not take too much time to take up the nurse's working hours.

(3)   Interaction

The process of effective communication must be interactive, not a process of transmitting information in one-way direction.

The information starts from the sender and arrives at the receiver. The sender needs to receive feedback and knows whether the information is understood and what effect is produced before the interaction can be completed. This is especially important in the process of medical communication in the clinic, it may be that the doctor has more contact with the patient.

However, for hospitalized patients, nurses spend much more time in contact with patients than doctors, and it is necessary to communicate effectively with patients. When asking a patient, try not to use closed questions, such as "yes" or "no". More open questions should be used, such as:

"What do you think?", "What do you feel?" To collect more detailed and extensive information, positive interaction and immediate feedback are also needed to encourage patients to make more statements.

Meanwhile, in communicating with patients, the nurse should interact with the patient to ensure that the patient understands the information and intentions. For example, the nurse tells the patient to take aspirin half an hour before breakfast. The patient may take it half an hour after breakfast. The nurse interacts with the patient during communication and asks when the aspirin is taken. Medical staff must ensure that the patient accurately understands the information.

3.2. *Summary*

In the nurse–patient communication, firstly, the nurse needs to listen to the patient or family members, try to let the patients and their families vent and confide, and explain the patient's condition as accurately as possible. Secondly, it is necessary to know the patient's examination results and treatment well, and the psychological pressure caused by medical expenses to the patient.

Thirdly, the nurse should pay attention to the educational level, emotional state and communicating feelings, the cognition of the condition, expectations, and the emotional response of the communication object. Nurses should learn to control themselves, and do not vent their bad emotions to the patient.

Also, the nurse should avoid using tone, intonation, and statements that stimulate the other person's emotions, avoid suppressing the other party's emotions, do not deliberately change the other's point of view, avoid using too many professional words that are not easy to understand, and avoid forcing the other party to accept the doctor's opinions and facts immediately.

Finally, the nurse should take the initiative to care, help, and patiently comfort the patient, take the initiative to inspect the ward, and actively send the patient out. If each nursing staff can communicate with the patient according to the above points, good nurse–patient communication effect would be achieved and good nurse–patient relationship would be established.

4. Skills of medical technician–patient communication

Medical technicians are the staff who use medical technology in a hospital, and they include the staff of medical laboratory, medical imaging (the doctor or the technician of the X-ray, CT, MRI), pharmacy (pharmacist clinical), medical function room (doctor or technician in ultrasound room, electrocardiogram room, gastrointestinal endoscopy room), pathology department (pathologist or pathology technician). Some of them are doctors, e.g., the doctor of radiology department reads the films and sends reports eventually; others are technicians such as X-ray photographers who assist doctors and nurses to collect the information of patients' diseases.

The technicians are ordinary technicians and do not have a doctor's license. While the doctors among medical technicians also have a lot of difference with general doctors because they do not give patients a diagnosis and treatment plan directly, and only give assistance in some way. Therefore, compared with doctors or nurses, medical technicians have less direct communication and contact with patients, but in the mind of patients, they may not be distinguished from doctors.

Therefore, the technician–patient communication also needs to follow the principles and skills of doctor–patient communication as explained in the second section.

The functions of medical technicians are relatively single, and they are only collecting information from a single field, so the time of communication with patients is extremely short. Because the purpose of communication between technicians and patients is extremely specific, patients would be more focused. Therefore, we would get better result of medical communication through technician–patient communication. At this time, medical communication should mainly focus on assistant medical care. Brochures and popular science videos should be taken into consideration while patients are waiting. Next, we will elaborate on different medical technicians.

4.1. *Medical laboratory staff*

Among medical technicians, medical inspectors can only contact patients when collecting blood, urine, and other specimens of patients. Most of the rest of the time, they deal with specimens and instruments. Therefore, the communication time with the patient is very short. But many patients are afraid of collecting specimens, especially blood specimens. They think collecting more blood samples may harm their health. In the test waiting area, staff can set some publicity columns to inform the patient about the points of attention when collecting blood samples and whether the collection of blood samples has any impact on the patient's health and relax the patient's emotions. Prepare some medical videos about reading test reports so that patients can watch and learn simple medical tests while waiting.

4.2. *Medical image staff*

Medical image staff include doctors and technicians. Technicians are mainly responsible for helping patients to take a medical picture. They also have direct contact with patients. The medical imaging department makes diagnosis with the images and do not contact with patients directly. Even with the technician, the time of contact with the patient may be very short, that is, a few minutes to 10 minutes during the filming process.

When the imaging department conducts medical communication, there are fewer opportunities for direct face-to-face communication with the patient. It may be more necessary to use propaganda manuals, videos, or content disseminated through we media, new media, etc. For example, which diseases could be diagnosed by medical imaging, whether medical imaging is harmful for the health, what are the differences between X-ray, CT, and MRI, and which imaging technique is more suitable for which disease.

4.3. *Staff in the function room*

Medical staff in the function room include the doctors and technicians who work in the ultrasound room, ECG, gastrointestinal endoscope room, etc. Ultrasound, ECG, and gastrointestinal endoscope are all the auxiliary examining methods in clinical diagnosis. They can provide referential suggestions for doctor's clinical diagnosis, but can't diagnose directly only according to the conclusions of the auxiliary examination. It still needs to be combined with the clinic to make an appropriate diagnosis. The medical staff in the function room have very short time to contact with the patient, and barely have a second chance or multiple chances to contact with patients. Some propaganda columns, brochures, and advertising videos can be made to put in the waiting area. For example, when the patient waits for a gastroscope, playing a gastroscope note in the gastroscope room, or a popular science video of what symptoms require a gastroscope examination, will receive a good result. When the function room doctor examines the patient, although the contact time is not long, they could also have some medical communication about the relevant examination. For instance, the ultrasound examination of breast found that patients with breast nodules usually need to pay attention to what they need to eat, how long it takes to re-examine, or what symptoms need to be treated in the hospital. These notes can all achieve good results.

4.4. *Staff in the pathology department*

The doctors and technicians in the pathology department also belong to medical staff. They usually deal with clinicians and pathological specimens, and barely get direct contact with patients. Furthermore, the reading and diagnosis of pathological specimens are very difficult and complicated, which need to combine with clinic examination, and the accuracy of pathological result is related to the quality of pathology collection. The medical communication of pathologists should be aimed more at those who are professional medical staff but are laymen in pathology than at ordinary people without medical knowledge.

4.5. *Clinical pharmacist*

Among medical staff, clinical pharmacists are different from other medical technicians.

Clinical pharmacists do not refer to the personnel who dispense drugs in hospital pharmacies, but a profession based on clinical pharmacy that combines medicine, discusses the law of clinical application of drugs, and implements rational drug utilization. As a profession, clinical pharmacist stems from the United States, and it is regarded as a newly emerging profession in China.

Clinical pharmacists use their rich knowledge of modern pharmacy to work with clinicians to design and provide the most reasonable and secure dosage schedule for patients.

A clinical pharmacist is a person who plays a key role in helping doctors use drugs properly. He can help doctors to prescribe the right drugs and dose at the right time to avoid bad interactions between drugs. To solve the problems encountered in factors related to drug treatment, nowadays, many hospitals have already set up the outpatient service for medicine consultation, which is taken care of by clinical pharmacists, in order to help patients in solving problems of using medicines. Clinical pharmacists are not clinical physicians, but their duties are connected with clinicians. At present, many patients suffer from a variety of diseases. The same patient may need to take a variety of drugs. Some patients may even have to take more than a dozen drugs every day. Multiple drugs are used at the same time; not only may there be interactions, but also side effects may occur. Clinical pharmacists can communicate some medical knowledge about the rational use of drugs in drug consultation clinics or other suitable occasions. The skill and precautions of clinical pharmacist–patient communication can be referred to in Section 2 of the physician–patient communication skill.

Chapter 5

Challenges and Countermeasures of Doctor–Patient Communication in the New Period

1. Status, challenges, and responses of doctor–patient communication

In recent years, violent conflicts between doctors and patients in China have exploded. Doctor–patient conflict refers to the behavior of both doctors and patients in the process of diagnosis and treatment, for their own interests, for some medical behaviors, methods, attitudes, and consequences, such as differences in cognition and understanding, resulting in violation of the legitimate rights and interests of the other party.[1] Poor communication and lack of trust are prominent features of the current Chinese doctor–patient relationship. Relative to the patient, the medical staff is more aware of this tension, and more than half of the medical staff believe that the doctor–patient relationship is "somewhat tense" or "very tense", but only a quarter of patients think so.

According to a survey conducted by the Chinese Medical Doctor Association, more than 90.1% of doctor–patient disputes are caused by improper communication. A recent survey of outpatient doctor–patient

---

[1] Liu, P. (2018). Investigation and countermeasures on the relationship between doctors and patients in outpatients. *Journal of Traditional Chinese Medicine Management, 26*(4), 9–11.

relationship shows that patients and medical staff have listed doctor–patient communication as one of the leading causes of tension of doctor–patient relationship.[2] How to communicate with patients and their families effectively and build a harmonious doctor–patient relationship, has become a clinical skill that every medical staff must possess. In 2002, the Accreditation Council for Graduate Education included the training of "interpersonal communication and communication skills and professionalism" in the six core occupational abilities of residents. According to the survey of residents in China, 92.2% think that it is necessary to conduct a doctor–patient communication skills course, integrate doctor–patient communication into the compulsory training course system for residents, and improve the communication skills of residents and patients, so that they have good professionalism and job competence.[3]

1.1. *The reasons for the tense doctor–patient relationship*

1.1.1. *The knowledge of the doctors and patients are not equal*

In the medical field, doctors are absolute authority, with rich medical knowledge and experience. A doctor has to undergo a period of formal medical theory education, practical operation, success and failure experience, thus forming a kind of understanding of the disease. Medical practitioners with special professional knowledge and skills are in an advantageous position. However, the popularization of medical knowledge in China is very weak, and the medical knowledge of the various groups and classes of society is generally lacking, and the patient group is in an uninformed disadvantage. Most of the patients are ordinary people, have no medical knowledge, or have very little medical knowledge. Some of the problems that are obvious in the eyes of doctors may be difficult to understand for the patients. The professional knowledge incompatibility

---

[2] Ibid.

[3] Shixian, G., Zhang, A., & Huo, G. (2018). Investigation on the status of communication between doctors and patients in a hospital affiliated to a hospital in Beijing. *Hospital Management Forum, 35*(1), 26–28, 45.

of doctors and patients may cause patients to blindly trust the doctors. Second, there is a lack of understanding. I listen to you because you know; I don't listen to you because I don't know, which is the patient's universal mindset. For doctors, because of their strong position, it is inevitable that there will be complaints about perfunctory sloppiness. I know what to say, and you don't know why you blame me. Because of the unequal knowledge obtained by the doctors and patients, if the doctors do not master certain methods and techniques, they may lead to misunderstandings and even contradictions between the doctors and patients when they communicate,

To give a simple example, a patient is sent to a hospital emergency room for acute cerebral infarction. The situation is quite critical. At this time, the doctor judges that the patient needs emergency thrombolysis, so the doctor talks with the patient's family and tells the patient's family that thrombolytic therapy is needed, informing them of the possible benefits of thrombolysis, also the possibility of inducing cerebral hemorrhage and ultimately leading to death. For the doctor, he tells the family about the possible treatment, the possible benefits and possible risks, but for the family members, they will feel that the risks of the patient, regardless of treatment or no treatment, are both very high. The doctor's words are equal to saying nothing. At this time, there is an inequality in the knowledge of both sides. If the treatment is not appropriate, it may cause contradictions between the doctors and the patients. The doctor should analyze the patient's specific situation to the family, including the benefits of active treatment and the possible risks, the benefits of non-active treatment and the possible risks, weighing the pros and cons, carefully analyzing, and then negotiating with the patient's family, making the most favorable and appropriate decisions for the patient.

For another example, every winter and spring is the high season of influenza. Influenza is an acute respiratory infection caused by seasonal influenza viruses. It is also a highly contagious and fast-transmitting disease. Influenza viruses are classified into three types: A, B, and C. The type A virus often undergoes antigenic variation, which is highly contagious, spreading rapidly, and is prone to widespread epidemics. Influenza viruses are mainly transmitted by droplets in the air, contact between people or contact with contaminated items. Typical clinical symptoms are: high fever, generalized pain, significant weakness, and mild respiratory symptoms, which can cause very serious complications, and may even lead to death. However, the common cold is a common acute upper respiratory viral infection, which is caused by rhinovirus, parainfluenza virus, respiratory syncytial virus, echovirus, coxsackie virus, coronavirus, adenovirus, and the like. Clinical manifestations include nasal congestion, sneezing, salivation, fever, cough, headache, and so on, which are mostly self-limiting. Most of them are distributed, multiple in winter and spring seasons, but there will be no pandemic. The symptoms of influenza and common cold are very similar at the beginning of the onset, may have fever, muscle soreness, cough, and other symptoms, but the flu may cause epidemics, and the common cold generally does not; relatively speaking, the symptoms of the common cold are mild which also cause less serious complications, but the flu may cause serious complications and even death. In the course of clinical diagnosis and treatment, patients or family members often ask: just getting a cold, how can it be so serious? How can it lead to the death of the patient? In fact, patients are likely to get influenza with complications occurring. Even in the common cold, some people with low immunity may get complications such as pneumonia and myocarditis, and eventually leading to death. Recently, an article was widely spread in the circle of friends: "Checking the influenza in the morning and passing away in the afternoon", saying that there is an elderly patient who has a cold-like symptom. The family thinks it is a common cold, and the doctor asks him to check the flu. But the family members did not think it was necessary, and in a short period of time, the patient died. The patient or family members are weak in medical knowledge, and it is indeed possible and qualified to question the patient's condition and the doctor's treatment. However, the doctor is a medical professional, in which case the medical principle needs to be popularized to the patient or his family, informing them of the difference between the flu and the common cold, and why the patient has complications, what complications have occurred, what are the hazards, making the patient or family members understand the disease and the progress of the disease clearly. With clear and good communication, doctor–patient conflicts would happen less frequently.

1.1.2. *The trend of materialization of doctor–patient relationship*

With the continuous advancement of medicine and development of high technology, a large number of high-end, sophisticated, and advanced instruments for medical use are constantly emerging, which are convenient for doctor's diagnosis and treatment, also reducing the chance of the direct face-to-face exchange and communication between doctors and patients. When a patient visits a doctor, the doctor often only looks at the patient's disease from a professional point of view and provides a series of tests that use various examination equipment to complete the diagnosis and treatment. Behind the rate of improving disease diagnosis and treatment is the "materialization" of the medical process. In modern times, many doctors have a high dependence on high-tech equipment during the diagnosis and treatment process, and neglect to communicate well with patients. The materialization of doctor–patient relationship reduces direct communication between the two sides, also weakens the feelings of both doctors and patients. Those high-end, sophisticated, and advanced medical machines not only separate the connection between doctors and patients, but also restrict the emotional and ideological communication between them. Under the trend of materialization of doctors and patients, doctors only pay attention to the disease itself, the disease and the sick are separated, the natural and social people, the physiological people and the people with thoughts and emotions are separated.

For example, if a patient's persistent headache cannot be alleviated, the doctor would recommend the patient do a series of examinations such as head CT, head MRI, EEG, 24-hour blood pressure monitoring after consultation, but neglecting that the patient's headache is relative to recent mental and work pressures and poor sleep, which can be found by carefully asking the patient's medical history. When the doctor relies too much on the equipment for diagnosis and treatment, the chance of communicating with the patient, asking for detailed medical history, establishning a good doctor–patient relationship is less, which is the adverse effect of the materialization of doctor–patient relationship.

In the state of material doctor–patient relationship, doctors would rely on equipment to diagnose too much. While reducing communication with patients, doctors' clinical diagnosis and treatment ability may also decline. Sometimes doctors can't even diagnose without high-end equipment, which may increase the medical expenses of patients improperly. For example, a patient goes to the hospital because of abdominal pain. After a simple inquiry about the medical history, the doctor asks the patient to do a gastroscopy to see what is wrong with the stomach, and then to make a colonoscopy to see what is wrong with the intestines, then to do an abdominal CT to see if there are any problems with the liver, gallbladder, and pancreas. If you can't find out any problem, you may need to have a small colonoscopy or the like. If it is a woman, you may have to do a gynecological ultrasound, and so on, the doctor may make several appointments related to abdominal pain, and the related medical expenses are also expensive. Of course, we can't deny that some abdominal pains are caused by very complicated reasons. Doctors do need to use some sophisticated equipment to confirm the diagnosis, but if the doctor needs to use sophisticated equipment to confirm the diagnosis to all patients, it would show that the doctor's ability is defective.

In the state of materialization of doctor–patient relationship, there is still a potential problem that cannot be ignored. Because of the worsening relationship between doctors and patients, in order to protect themselves doctors have to do a lot of related inspections to confirm their diagnosis. For example, a patient came to the hospital because of a stuffy nose for two days, no fever, no cough, and no other accompanying symptoms; the doctor gave him a throat examination and a lung auscultation which were both negative, and there were no special symptoms in the throat examination, no abnormal breath sounds, and voices in the lungs. The doctor judged that the patient might be getting an ordinary cold, so gave him some cold medicine and asked him to take a good rest. After a few days, the patient developed cough and fever, so went to the hospital again and found that it was pneumonia, so the patient began to question why the doctor did not give him a chest radiograph at the first time. He began to make big noises and demand compensation. In fact, this is a normal development process of the disease. The doctor who first accepted the patient did not have any medical errors. However, because the patient strongly demanded, the doctor finally compensated. However, the doctor may have a chest radiograph for all similar patients at the onset of the disease to avoid disputes between doctors and patients later, which is actually an overkill and will worsen doctor–patient relationship to form a vicious circle.

1.1.3. *The issue of doctor's attitude*

After graduating from a medical school, medical students must go through a long training course and pass numerous exams before they can become a real doctor. Because the training period is quite long, the training experience is quite difficult and complicated, those who can become doctors are the best among their peers. For this reason, some doctors will have a certain sense of pride, and there will be a sense of superiority in the face of patients. At the same time, as most doctors are full or even overloaded with work, some doctors think that it is a waste of time to communicate with patients. In the face of patients, they will be indifferent and eager to send patients away, which is easy to cause dissatisfaction of patients.

For instance, a patient has traveled from a remote mountainous area for a long time to a famous hospital. He has been queuing since the early hours of the morning and finally registered with the expert number of a reputable doctor, and then lined in the waiting area for one day, and finally it was his turn to see a doctor. If the doctor was only cold-hearted and rushed to send the patient, this would inevitably cause a strong complaint from the patient, because it was not easy for him to come once and he hoped to get the expert's careful diagnosis and treatment. Although doctors are quite busy with their work, and hardly have a lot of time for consultation, if they are able to be attentive and amiable at the time of admission, focusing on the patient's problems in a short period of time, or give the patients some suggestions, the patients are less likely to have dissatisfaction, and the communication between doctors and patients will be much smoother.

To give another example, a patient has a malignant tumor. Because of his very young age, the doctor suggests that he should be actively treated. The family refuses, so the doctor is very angry and teaches the family members of the patient a lesson, resulting in contradictions between the two sides. The doctor thinks that his advice is absolutely correct, how can such a young patient give up active treatment? However, there may be other deep-seated reasons behind the family's refusal to receive treatment. For example, their family is in great financial difficulties. In addition to this patient, there is also a patient who is in bed for a long time in the family. There is simply no way to afford medical care and no one to take care of the patients. If the doctor can not only treat the disease, but also pay more attention to the problems behind the disease, instead of putting himself in a position of absolute authority, he can understand the patients and their families better, and the communication between them will be better and smoother.

1.1.4. *The issue of patient's attitude*

Most of the patients are ordinary people without basic medical knowledge. Once they get sick, they may feel uneasy or even irritated due to the lack of relevant knowledge. At the same time, some patients simply consider the hospital as a service industry, the doctor is selling (or providing) labor with rich knowledge, experience, and technology, the patient is buying a labor product — health, so they will think that as long as they pay with the money, the hospital should cure all the diseases, and also some patients will think that only if they go to the hospital, they will be cured no matter what disease they get. If the effect is not satisfactory, it is the problem of the hospital and the doctor. Many patients spend money on medical treatment, just like going to a shopping mall to repair a TV set. No matter how many parts are included, how much science and technology is involved, and how complicated the repair needs to be, he does not need to know. He just needs to be able to take it home and watch it. When seeing a doctor, he also does not care how the doctor uses technology, how hard it is, as it is the doctor's business. They only want to cure the disease finally, and they believe that the disease can be cured with money, just as the TV set can be fixed with money. What they don't know is that even a TV set, if it breaks down, won't always be fixed and will eventually be scrapped. Nor do they know the limitation that some diseases, in the field of medicine, are still incurable. The famous saying of American doctor Trudo, "sometimes, to heal; often, to help; always, to comfort", is a visual illustration of the situation; due to the particularity and complexity of medicine, "cure" is "sometimes", not "often", not "always", and hospitals are not shops you can spend money to buy health and life, as human life and health are priceless. Some patients bring their dissatisfaction in other fields to medical institutions. They simply think that hospitals are for making money, and also for interpersonal relationships. Without interpersonal relationships, they cannot be hospitalized. They do not respect doctors and do not follow the necessary rules of hospitals. They lack the basic qualities of being patients or responsible ordinary people.

For example, the emergency department of the hospital is generally open 24 hours a day, and the patient can go to the doctor at any time, but the emergency treatment rule is: in any case, priority is given to critically ill patients. For example, there is a young patient who has a fever with a temperature of 38.5°C, no other accompanying symptoms, and the patient is in good condition generally. The emergency pre-examination nurse initially judges that it is a flat patient, and asks him to queue up for treatment in the emergency department of the hospital. At the same time, there is a senior citizen whose abdominal pain was severe and he was restless. The nurse arranges him to see a doctor before the young patient. The young patient is dissatisfied and makes a big noise, causing doctor–patient conflicts. In fact, he does not know that according to the classification of the emergency department, the old man has been graded to a higher level, which means that the condition is more critical, and he is at a relatively low level, the condition is relatively stable, and should be treated after the elderly patient. The rules of emergency care have never been first come, first served, but critical patients first in all countries. This young patient not only does not have the basic qualities of general public humility, nor does he follow the good quality of hospital rules during treatment. When he quarreled with the hospital, it would not only affect his own medical treatment, but also affect the treatment of the critically ill old man, which is very immoral behavior.

For example, a young male patient who took a medical insurance card from his mother came to see a doctor because he did not have medical insurance. The doctor found that he was using another person's medical insurance card, not only his age was wrong, but also his gender was not right, so he admitted. The doctor refused to see him using a fraudulent identity and asked him to register in his own capacity. The patient shouted, saying that the doctor's attitude was not good. This is a typical unreasonable trouble and should be condemned.

1.1.5. *Dishonesty between doctors and patients*

Both doctors and patients need to abide by the principle of good faith. The doctor's integrity lies in the need to communicate and inform patients based on medical guidelines, which cannot be exaggerated. The patient's integrity lies in telling the doctor all the medical history which cannot be concealed or deceived, so that the doctor can carry out necessary diagnosis and treatment.

For example, a patient admitted to the ward because of poor glycemic control due to diabetes concealed his history of open tuberculosis. Because he concealed his medical history, doctors admitted him to the general ward without special protective measures. During his stay in hospital, because his tuberculosis is contagious, he is likely to transmit it to the medical staff who helped him and other patients in the same ward. This is a typical case of the patient's dishonesty, which may affect the patient himself, but also may bring harm to other patients and medical staff.

To give another example, in order to defraud sick leave, a patient complained of high fever and went to the hospital to ask for a doctor. After the nurse gave him a thermometer, the patient put it in his own hot water cup. The nurse checked the thermometer and found his body temperature was really high, so he was arranged to the emergency department. The emergency doctors found that the patient was generally in good condition, without symptoms and signs corresponding to high fever which was so different. So the patient was asked to re-test the body temperature and carry out a series of tests. The patient refused examination and refused to use all drugs, only asked for sick leave, causing contradictions between the two sides. In the case of some patients concealing their medical history, some patients also describe the diseases they do not have as their own diseases. They only intend to take sick leave or prescribe drugs for other people in the family, and some patients may even sell prescribed drugs to second-hand dealers. which is not only a matter of good faith, but also has the possibility of fraudulently obtaining medical insurance funds or breaking the law.

There was once a man who loaned his medical insurance card to his brother. Because they two are similar in age and appearance, his brother used his medical insurance card to see a doctor. At first, the medical staff did not find the problem of fraudulent use. However, because his brother was critically ill, he died shortly after admission. The medical staff issued a death certificate based on the patient's medical information. At this time, the man discovered a serious problem because he lent his health insurance card to his brother. He was considered "dead", but in fact he was still alive. So he needs to prove through various ways that he is not dead. This is also an unexpected and very serious consequence of dishonesty in medical treatment.

From the perspective of the doctor's integrity, for example, a patient came to the hospital for pain due to lumbar pain and numbness of both lower extremities. The doctor judged the patient to have lumbar disc herniation after examination, because the symptoms of the patient were already obvious, and seriously affected normal life. Doctors recommend surgery: before the operation, the doctor should inform the patient about the success rate of surgical treatment, what complications may occur, if the doctor tells the patient that the success rate of surgery is 100% and there is no possibility of any complications, then it is an exaggeration and a manifestation of the doctor's dishonesty, which may mislead the patient's treatment options and prognosis.

1.1.6. *Communication between the doctors and patients is behind time*

Most patients are ordinary people without medical knowledge, and their understanding of medicine is mostly from doctors' notification and communication. Therefore, the doctors are not only responsible for treating the sick and saving people, but also responsible for communicating with the patients and their families. Some medical staff have insufficient understanding of the importance of doctor–patient communication. They have not realized the importance of strengthening communication between doctors and patients, improving "patient-centered" humanized services, improving the quality of medical services, establishing hospital brands, and building a harmonious relationship between doctors and patients. In the past, many medical colleges in China mainly borrowed the medical education model of the former Soviet Union, partially culti-vating medical skills and ignoring communication education. In terms of curriculum, doctor–patient communication skills training is basically blank in undergraduate and postgraduate education in medical colleges. There is no special curriculum, and even if these courses are offered, the content is simple and not very practical, and as an elective course, stu-dents can only master some basic knowledge, and often face embarrass-ing situations in clinical internships and medical activities. Because there is no special training in doctor–patient communication, many doctors do not know how to communicate well with patients, nor do they think that communication is an important method to establish a harmonious rela-tionship between doctors and patients. Some doctors believe that com-munication between doctors and patients is a waste of time, which is very wrong.

In exchange and communication, in addition to paying attention to the accuracy of the content of communication, we must also pay attention to the timing of communication. Timely and effective communication can bring good experience to both doctors and patients; without timely or even after-the-fact communication, sometimes this may cause unnecessary misunderstandings or contradictions between the two parties.

For example, a patient underwent surgery for a thyroid nodule and a frozen section during surgery revealed that the nodule was malignant in nature, which is known as thyroid cancer in the traditional sense. At this time, it is necessary for the surgeon to send professionals to communicate with the patient's family immediately and change the plan to expand the scope of surgical cleaning. After obtaining the understanding and authori-zation of the family, the surgeon can change the surgical method; but if the surgeon does not immediately communicate with the family, but first change the surgical plan and scope of surgery according to the situation found during the operation, and then informs the patient after the opera-tion, this is not a timely communication in the doctor–patient relationship, and it is likely to cause dissatisfaction of the patient's family members. For family members, they have the right to know the patient's condition, but also the right to discuss with the doctor and jointly decide on the treat-ment plan for the patient.

1.1.7. *Defective communication between doctors and patients*

Doctors and patients are strangers who are not familiar with each other and they are connected because of patients or diseases. Therefore, when the two parties communicate, they may not be as tacit as family or familiar people. If one party adopts a more blunt communication method, it may cause misunderstandings or contradictions between the two sides.

Doctor–patient communication is divided into language communication and non-verbal communication. Language is a convention system of symbols, a psychological process in which humans exchange ideas and express emotions. The exchange of ideas and communication through linguistic symbols is the essential feature of human beings and the premise and basis for the interaction between doctors and patients. As a tool for communication activities, most of the interpersonal interactions are achieved through language. In other words, if the patient's inner world is an unknown one, the doctor's language is the bridge to the other side. If inappropriate language communication is used, both doctors and patients may have misunderstandings and even contradictions. The same is true for non-verbal communication. If a doctor receives a patient and always adopts an indifferent face, the attitude toward the patient is also ignored, and it is easy to cause disputes between the two parties.

For example, a doctor who has been in the outpatient clinic has been working for a long time and needs to go to the toilet. When it is the turn of a patient, he tells the patient that he has something to do and asks the patient to wait for a while. The patient was very angry. He waited for so long. When it was his turn, the doctor had something to do, so he said excitedly: No, how can the doctor have other things? You have to finish my illness before you can do other things. This has caused contradictions between doctors and patients. From the patient's point of view, the patient's mood is very anxious. In order to see a doctor, it may involve a leave of absence or long-distance travel. The time is limited. Of course, the patients hope to get the doctor's diagnosis and treatment as soon as possible. In terms of the doctors, he has been working in the clinic for so long. It is reasonable to go to the toilet, and how could he not get the patient's   understanding?   If   the   two   sides   change   the   way   of communication, the doctor informs the other party of his intention to go to the toilet and tells him that he has been working in the clinic for a long time, and will return as soon as possible, it is easier to get the patient's understanding. If the patient knows that the doctor has been working for a few hours, and even has no time for a toilet break, he will understand the doctor well and be willing to wait in the clinic.

For another example, when a patient comes to consult a doctor if he could stop medication, the doctor feels that this is not appropriate, and he is very blunt to say to the patient: Are you a doctor or am I a doctor? Listen to you or listen to me? Such words are very strong and do not respect the patients themselves, and it is easy to cause contradictions and conflicts between the two sides. Both doctors and patients should be in an equal relationship, rather than the doctor being at a high level, and the patient having to yield to it. If the doctor can improve the communication method at this time and inform the patient that it is inappropriate to stop the drug treatment currently as it will cause a lot of complications, and the patient still needs to follow the doctor's advice and take the medicine on time, the patient will be more likely to accept the doctor's advice. Good communication with both sides thinking about each other is very beneficial to improve doctor–patient relationship and avoid doctor–patient conflicts.

1.1.8. *The doctor's communication content is inconsistent*

Medical behavior is not a single individual's behavior. It needs to be done in the form of teamwork. For example, a surgery, in addition to the surgeon, requires the first assistant, second assistant, anesthesiologist, and surgical nurse to assist. In other medical treatments, doctors from different departments and levels are often required to make joint decisions. If the doctors in different departments have different interpretations during the whole process of treatment, it will cause doubts for the patients, and they will even think that the doctor is perfunctory and deceiving himself.

For example, a patient came to see a small nodule in the lungs. At this time, the doctor of the respiratory medicine told him not to worry, the follow-up would be fine, but the doctor of the thoracic surgery told him that surgery was necessary, otherwise it is very possible to be malignant. Two different doctors put forward completely different opinions, and it is bound to cause doubts.

Another example is an elderly patient hospitalized with pulmonary infection. One doctor told his family that the patient was very serious because he was older and had heart failure. Another doctor told the family that it was just a common pneumonia, and there was no need to worry too much. He could be discharged in a few days. Different interpretations from different doctors will inevitably make the patients' families feel that the treatment team is unprofessional and there is no communication and coordination between them. For the medical team, every member of the team represents the team. If it is needed to explain the patient's condition, it is necessary to communicate and maintain consistency in advance. Otherwise, it is easy to mislead the patient. For some patients with complex conditions, unknown etiology and difficult treatment, multi-department consultation can be considered to give a consensus opinion, so as to avoid inconsistency in the interpretation of patients. Here, it should also be pointed out that "doctor" in doctor–patient communication refers not only to doctors, but also to medical groups such as nurses, medical technicians, managers, and logisticians. As long as they are members of the medical team, whether as doctors, nurses, medical technicians, or others, they should be consistent when communicating with patients. If not, it can be clarified after discussion in the team. As long as they are members of the medical team or the hospital, the patients think that they represent the hospital. If two hospital members say something inconsistent, the patients will have a lot of questions.

Sometimes the content of communication between doctors and patients is inconsistent because of the progress of the patient's disease. For example, a patient with hypertension had limb weakness and recovered quickly. No problem was found in the cranial CT examination. According to the patient's medical history, physical examination and the report of the cranial CT examination, the doctor judged that the patient was suffering from transient ischemic attack and gave the corresponding treatment. One day later, the patient had hemiplegia on one side of the limb. The review of the cranial CT clearly indicated that the patient was suffering from cerebral infarction. The occurrence of these conditions is actually caused by the progress of the patient's disease. But for patients and their families, the same doctor told them different conditions in the first two days and it may be difficult to understand. At this time, doctors need to be patient and explain in detail to the patients or their families why this happened, what treatment methods are available so that the patients and their families can clearly understand the origin of the situation, so that the doctor–patient contradiction will not easily arise. If the doctor only informs the patient without explaining and informing the original cause, it will easily lead to misunderstanding between the two sides.

1.1.9. *The patient's rights and legal awareness have been strengthened*

In the continuous advancement of society, the people's legal awareness is also constantly strengthening, which is very commendable for the progress of social legalization. However, medicine is still a science that needs to be explored so far, that is to say, in many medical fields, there are still many unsolved mysteries, and there are still no good treatments for many diseases. It is the right of the patients to defend their rights in a reasonable area, but it is debatable if the patient's rights are beyond the basic principles and principles of medicine.

For example, a patient who went to hospital because of progressive muscle weakness, went through several hospitals, and finally got a diagnosis of motor neuron disease in a famous hospital. This is an incurable disease, and patients will gradually develop the emergence of muscle atrophy, until the death due to respiratory failure. Modern medicine does not have a good treatment, and can only support the treatment of disease and prolong life. If the family members protect their rights because of delay in the diagnosis and go to complain or sue the first few hospitals that fail to make a definitive diagnosis at this time, it is an excessive act of rights protection to a certain extent, because the diagnosis of this disease is unanimously recognized.

To give another example, a car accident patient was very critical when he was sent to the hospital. At the end of the day, even though with the doctor's active rescue, the patient eventually died. At this time, the patient's family told the court that the doctor's treatment was improper and not timely, ignoring that the cause of the patient's death is actually a serious car accident, believing that as long as the person is still alive when he is sent to the hospital, the hospital must rescue the patient. This is a typical over-protection. To a certain extent, the cause of excessive rights protection is because the patients or their families do not understand the uncertainty of medicine, but if the excessive rights are frequent, it will seriously hurt the doctor's enthusiasm for treating patients.

Let us give examples of the rights that some patients have. The law stipulates that patients have the right to know. Many patients use this right. Of course, most patients use the right properly, but some patients may cause contradictions between doctors and patients if the rights are overused or improperly used.

1.2. *The patient's right to know*

1.2.1. *The right to know the condition*

The right to know the condition means that the patient has the right to know his or her health information, to understand the true situation and development trend of the disease, and the medical staff must not conceal any information related to the patient's health. However, according to Article 11 of the Medical Accident Treatment Regulations, medical personnel can weigh the physical and mental conditions of patients according to specific conditions and selectively inform patients about the condition. Its purpose is to create a good psychological environment for patients, which is conducive to maintaining the stability of the patient's condition and providing better conditions for treatment. However, the patient's actual condition must be informed to the patient's family, which is unconditional. For example, an elderly patient has advanced tumors, and the doctor informed the patient's family members of the condition, and then according to the request of the patient's family, did not inform the patient, hoping not to bring too much mental burden to the patient. One day, the patient inadvertently found out his condition, complaining that the doctor violated his right to know. At this time, after careful analysis it is thought that the doctor did not violate the patient's right to know, because the doctor has clearly informed the patient's family, then the patient was concealed in good faith under the patient's family's request. At this time, if there is a contradiction between the two sides, it should be better communicated, so that patients understand the ins and outs of the matter.

1.2.2. *The right to know the treatment measures*

The right to know the treatment means that the patient has the power to know the treatment measures for the patient to treat the disease in order to avoid and reduce the risk and has the right to choose to accept or refuse; the doctor is obliged to provide patients with various effective treatment plans for the disease and explain the pros and cons of various programs to the patients objectively and to inform all the links and contents of all kinds of treatment measures to the patients truthfully and realistically. Patients can weigh the pros and cons of the doctor's recommendation and choose the treatment that they think the best. The doctor must respect the patient's choices and do his best to implement the patient's choice of treatment. For example, a patient has acute appendicitis. The doctor recommends surgery. The patient refuses and asks for conservative treatment. After communicating with the doctor, he agrees to conservative treatment, but it is necessary to observe the condition closely. However, after conservative treatment, the patient's condition continues to deteriorate. Appendicitis developed into an appendix abscess and was eventually treated with surgery. At this time, the patient complained that the doctor did not inform him of the complexity of the condition and had doubts about the right to know about the treatment. However, in this case, the doctor actually fulfilled the patient's right to know about the treatment. The preferred treatment plan has been informed. On the one hand, the patient refuses the first treatment plan, and after using the second treatment plan, the patient's condition is also closely observed, and the treatment plan is changed in time when the condition changes; in this case, the patient's right is clearly over-utilized, or is used improperly.

1.2.3. *Medical expenses are known*

That means the patient and his relatives have the right to know the medical expenses, that is, the patient has the right to control the amount, use and expenditure progress of various medical expenses that he should bear for medical treatment. The medical department shall strictly implement relevant laws and regulations and departmental rules and regulations, and truthfully provide patients with information on medical expenses required. The doctor should select appropriate medical equipment and medicine according to the actual condition of the patient, and provide appropriate medical services, which can only be used after obtaining the consent of the patients and their relatives. For example, depending on the patient's condition, a certain drug needs to be used. This drug has two different manufacturers: one is imported and the price is relatively expensive, and the other is domestically produced and the price is relatively cheap. When the doctor uses it, he should inform the patient of the two different choices, so that the patient can clearly understand the choice, so contradictions between doctors and patients are less likely to occur.

When there are obstacles or even contradictions in the communication between doctors and patients, we should realize that this must not be a unilateral problem. To a large extent, both sides have certain problems. Then, when encountering problems, both sides need to calmly and carefully analyze the reasons for the misunderstandings and contradictions between the two sides, and then seek appropriate solutions for the reasons, avoiding the attitude of bluntness and anxiety, so that most of the problems can be solved. Of course, the first prerequisite for solving the problem is that both sides have a good attitude and hope to improve communication and exchanges between the two parties. If either party does not have a cooperative attitude, then it will not be able to solve the problems faced.

In addition, the authoritative media, as well as doctors, when communicating with patients, must also popularize the scientific nature of medicine, so that more people understand medicine and understand the limitations of medicine, while also understanding doctors and the doctors' efforts. Only when the two sides can achieve mutual respect, mutual understanding, mutual cooperation, mutual communication, and discussion, can the doctor–patient relationship become better and more harmonious. This is also the concept that medical communication needs to be spread and popularized at the level of "the concept of medicine". Let the ordinary people have an objective and rational "concept of medicine", which is the purpose of medical communication.

2. The "Dr. Internet" phenomenon and responding measures

By the end of 2017, China had 722 million internet users and internet penetration had achieved 55.8%.[4] Since "internet +" was first proposed in government work report by prime minister Li Ke Qiang in 2015, internet industry application of our country has been widely applied in all aspects of people's life, especially "internet + medical", which has made great headway. However, internet's extensive application brings obvious changes to traditional doctor–patient communication, and even affects doctor–patient relationship in the consulting room. The distinguished scholar J. Garry has asserted that the extensive application of internet will overturn traditional doctor–patient relationship, and the patient will replace doctor as the center of the medical service system in the 21st century.[5] According to the report on search behavior of Chinese netizens' science popularization needs, which was published by Science Popularization Department of China Association for Science and Technology, Baidu Brand Data Center and China Science Popularization Research Institute, in 2017, the top three popular science topics searched by Chinese citizens are: Health & medical care, IT, and aerospace. Health and medical care accounted for 63.16% of searches on eight topics which ranked the first; information technology-related searches ranked second with 11.05%; aerospace-related searches accounted for 6.00% of the total. The rankings of popular science topic search index in 2017 are health & medical, aerospace, cutting-edge technology, food

---

[4] http://www.cnnic.com.cn/hlwfzyj/hlwxzbg/hlwtjbg/201803/P020180305409870339136.pdf.
[5] Gary, J. (2006). *Clever patient* (Y. Qin & J. L. Tang, Trans.). Beijing: Peking University Medical Press.

safety, climate and environment, energy utilization, emergency risk avoidance, and IT. Comparing with the data in 2016, the following topics have increased growth ranking: health and medical, aerospace, cutting-edge technology, and food safety. In all searches, health and medical content is No. 1 indisputably, which has a clear gap from the No. 2 topic, and the growth rate is No.1 too. It can be seen that Chinese netizens are quite concerned about health and medical treatment, which also indicates that it has become a very popular trend and method to obtain health and medical knowledge through the internet.

There is no denying that extensive access to medical health knowledge on the internet will disrupt the old doctor paternalistic diagnosis model. Recent surveys have shown that three-quarters of Chinese patients get health information online.[6] Patients are more likely to track their own cutting-edge knowledge of the disease. Because doctors are dealing with multiple diseases and large amounts of data, patients only need to focus on one or more health concerns. Especially for patients with rare diseases and their families, their knowledge of this specific disease can even exceed that of the general doctor. Therefore, the traditional authority of medical workers has been greatly challenged. At the same time, because the internet information standard has many problems now, a lot of information is mixed with false information, even rumors. Ordinary patients have difficulty distinguishing right from wrong. Under such circumstances, how can medical personnel conduct medical communication effectively?

First of all, keep an open mind. Although most patients keep enough respect for the doctor, the present doctor–patient relationship is no longer about doctors telling their patients what do to. Patients may have searched on the internet for information about their conditions before entering the clinic. When a doctor's description does not match the results of his own search, many patients question it. Rather than seeing this as a challenge to their authority, medical staff should keep an open mind, and acknowledge patients' efforts and sort out their doubts. If it turns out that patients are

---

[6] Dai, F., Liu, Y., & Su, Y. (2014). Investigation of patient health information acquisition and medical service utilization under the network environment. *Journal of Medical Postgraduate, 27*(5), 1087–1110.

not getting the right information, doctors can take the opportunity to do a little medical science popularization.

Secondly, in addition to formal academic search, doctors also need to regularly search information from the perspective of ordinary people to see what kind of information is provided on the internet, so as to "know yourself and the enemy" and calmly deal with patients' doubts.

From the perspective of the search focus of general netizens on health content, there are also some regional differences. For example, netizens in northern China pay more attention to cardiovascular diseases, while those in southern China pay more attention to infectious diseases. There are also differences in time and season. For example, in winter and spring, netizens may pay more attention to diseases such as influenza and cardiovascular and cerebrovascular diseases, while in summer, they may pay more attention to intestinal infectious diseases and heat stroke. The searching contents about health can be mainly divided into three categories: disease diagnosis and treatment, hospitals, and health care knowledge.

Let's look at some simple examples and analyze them.

A patient came to the hospital with left chest pain. Beforehand, the patient checked on the Internet and concluded that nine times out of ten he had had a myocardial infarction, or at least angina. It is typical to search the diagnosis and treatment of diseases through the Internet. After arriving at the hospital and after detailed examination, the doctor discovered that the patient had not got the disease of the heart, but the chest pain was caused by shingles. At this point, the patient might not understand and thought the doctor was ignoring his own heart problems which might delay diagnosis and treatment. So at this time, on the one hand, the doctor could give the patient an electrocardiogram examination through which the doctor could tell the patient that the heart had no problem. On the other hand, the doctor could do some science popularization about chest pain and tell the patient that not all chest pains are caused by heart disease, and many diseases can cause chest pain. At the same time, the doctor needed to affirm that the patient's attitude of coming to hospital for chest pain was positive and correct. Through interaction and communication between the two sides, doctors can correct the partial medical knowledge that patients get from the Internet.

Again for instance, a patient recently had some stool bleeding. He searched on the Internet and read some medical information. According to the researched information, he decided he might have bowel cancer and went to the hospital for help. It is also a behavior of searching for the information about diagnosis and treatment of diseases through the Internet. The doctor inquired the patient's medical history in detail and gave him a thorough examination, from which the doctor found the patient did not develop bowel cancer, just a common hemorrhoid. However, the patient was still unable to dispel his doubts. At this time, in the process of communication with the patient, the doctor found that the patient had the idea of bowel cancer because recently a friend of his age died of advanced bowel cancer. Therefore he began to worry that he had the same disease after bleeding stool. On the one hand, doctors can popularize relevant knowledge after knowing the reasons behind it, inform the patient what disease can cause bleeding stool, what to notice and the symptoms of bowel cancer. On the other hand, according to the patient's panic, the doctor can do some psychological counseling and emotional relief. In the communication with patients, doctors can establish a good doctor–patient relationship, and gradually help the patient to establish a correct understanding of his own problems and unknown diseases.

When Internet users search for the diagnosis and treatment of diseases, they often search for some hospitals that treat diseases. Because a lot of people don't know which hospital is famous and which disease the hospital is famous for, the easiest way to know is to search on the Internet, comparing which hospital is the best, and go to that hospital. But searching on the Internet for hospitals is likely to get wrong information. For example, the case of Wei Zexi in 2016 is a typical one. Wei Zexi developed synovial sarcoma in 2014, which is a soft tissue malignancy that has yet to be treated. Through an internet search, his family found that a hospital in Beijing could conduct biological immune therapy with a high cure rate. So his family spent a fortune and took him to this hospital in Beijing for four courses of biologic immunotherapy, but he didn't see the expected results. Finally, Wei Zexi died. Later, his family learned that the hospital's so-called biological immunotherapy had been discontinued for use in foreign countries and had not been approved for use in China. Although the hospital was a public hospital, the clinic he was treated in was an informal unit contracted out to private practice, and its online ranking was bought. From this, we can see that the search on the Internet is not reliable in many cases. The ranking of some search engines is related to profits and money, which does not represent the actual ranking of the hospital. When the country and the law gradually purify the Internet environment, we also need to popularize to the public. If we need to search for the ranking of hospitals, we should search for the ranking given by regular institutions. For example, since 2010, the Hospital Management Institute of Fudan University has launched the "ranking list of hospital reputation in China" and "ranking list of Chinese hospitals" every year. The ranking project is a non-profit project conducted by an independent third party hospital management academic institution. Through the ranking and evaluation, it is beneficial to establish a benchmark for the discipline construction of the hospital and benefit the patients, helping to highlight the domestic and international reputation of the hospital specialty. Considering the value and significance of guiding patients to seek medical treatment regionally, more hospitals should be promoted to enter the public and patients' visions. The evaluation experts of the ranking are from the Chinese medical association and the physician association. The evaluation is very objective, and the ranking of famous hospitals and departments in China has been widely recognized, which can be referred to by patients. Therefore, when spreading medical knowledge to the public, it is also very necessary to teach the public to reasonably use the Internet to search for medical resources.

With the progress of society and economic development, many people have begun to pay attention to Health Preservation and Healthcare. Health Preservation and Healthcare refer to the maintenance of health, as well as the nourishing of life on the principle of adjusting Yin and Yang, harmonizing Qi and blood, spiritual self-cultivation, using many methods such as regulating the spirit, guiding the breath, health maintenance in four seasons, nourishing food, nourishing medicine, tempering desire, and inedia to achieve the goal of health and longevity. The easiest way to acquire health knowledge is the Internet and media. However, the information of health preservation on the Internet is intermingled, which makes it difficult to guarantee its authenticity and validity. At the same time, the general public is also unable to judge the accuracy of such knowledge, and is easy to be misled. On the one hand, there is a lot of fake and unreliable health knowledge on the Internet and media, such as the famous Zhang Wuben event in the past few years. Zhang Wuben was without medical background, but he packaged himself as a health care expert, famous for "the first food therapy in traditional Chinese medicine", and promoted his health care ideas in various media platforms. The most famous of these is the mung bean health concept and "Eat Out the Diseases You Have Eaten". He claimed that mung beans could treat lung cancer, diabetes, cardiovascular disease, pneumonia, and dozens of common difficult diseases, so that the price of mung beans rose and the beans even became out of stock. These health concepts are now proven to have no scientific basis, but in those days they affected many ordinary people. Zhang also spread some wrong health concepts, such as eating more salt is better, and there is already a lot of medical evidence linking excessive salt intake with high blood pressure. Zhang Wuben was still propagating this wrong idea, which actually brings immeasurable potential harm to many people. On the other hand, even if the health knowledge on the Internet is true, but whether it is suitable for themselves, ordinary people do not have the ability to identify and judge. For example, there is knowledge about exercise health on the Internet. It is suggested that people should have half an hour of aerobic exercise, 5 to 7 days a week, which can strengthen their bodies and reduce weight. This is true for the general population, but many people don't know what kind of exercise is aerobic exercise. Taking it a step further, it's worth discussing whether such exercises are suitable for everyone. If a patient has a cardiovascular disease, such as angina, then his exercise tolerance must be reduced, as improper exercise is likely to cause angina, or even lead to myocardial infarction and death. Even the correct knowledge of health care also needs to be clear about its beneficiaries. However, this judgment ability is not available to ordinary people, and it needs to be informed and cleared by medical personnel with professional knowledge. Therefore, when facing the concept of health preservation spread by the Internet, medical personnel should not only inform patients whether the concept is correct, but also tell patients whether the concept is suitable for a specific individual.

It should be said that the development of the Internet is in line with the trend of the era. And with the continuous development of smartphones and electronic networks, the number of internet users and the frequency of health-related content searching through the Internet will increase more and more in the future. On the one hand, when facing the internet doctors, we need to handle problems rationally; it is suggested to purify the network environment and screen out those false information. On the other hand, we need to shoulder the responsibility to distinguish the correct information from the incorrect information, and to help patients to get accurate medical knowledge from the internet doctor and to spread and disseminate appropriate and correct health knowledge. In the 2017 China Netcom Popular Science Needs Search Behavior Report, the top three occupations of the Chinese netizen science popularization groups are education, IT communication electronics, and medical and health. Among the popular science groups, the education industry accounted for the highest proportion, reaching 13.0%, followed by IT communication electronics, accounting for 9.8%. The proportion of medical and health professionals in the popular science group was 7.71%, which was significantly higher than that of all netizens (7.33%). According to the network information behavior of Chinese netizens, the main interest areas are divided. Information, medical health, and education and training are in the top three, and each proportion of groups is more than 10%. It can be seen that many medical workers have joined the army of network medical science spontaneously. While the network science is increasing, we all hope to further standardize the medical network science and ensure the quality and reliability, to avoid another tragedy like Wei Zexi.

3. The "Dr. Grandma" phenomenon and responding measures

Unlike the "internet doctors" relying on advanced network technology, the "Dr. Grandma" phenomenon reflects the challenges brought by traditional health concepts. The folk medical wisdom of our country has a long history and played a certain role in the long history. However, many backward unscientific health concepts are still plaguing people's daily lives. For example, in recent years, the "Houyuezi Heatstroke", which has been frequently reported, is a vivid example. This rare "heatstroke calving" in Europe and the United States is a disease with Chinese characteristics, which is related to the traditional "confinement" custom. Such traditional customs are mostly passed down from generation to generation, so this phenomenon is called the "Dr. grandma" phenomenon. Such patients or related family members are elderly groups who are likely to experience empirical interventions in disease treatment after accumulating certain life experiences. In the face of such a grandmother doctor phenomenon, medical staff can take the opportunity to carry out the relative medical communication and correct the misconceptions.

Here are some simple examples.

In the past three months of summer, a young patient couldn't eat food and lost his appetite and weight. An elder family member comforted him that this was a common phenomenon in the summer called "summer non-acclimatization" and he would be fine when getting some drugs which promote digestion. So after going to the hospital, the patient thought he was overexamined as the doctor asked him to have a gastroscopy. However, the doctor was so responsible that after inquiring about the medical history in details and giving the patient a complete physical examination, he repeatedly persuaded the patient to undergo a gastroscopy. Finally, the patient agreed. The gastroscopic indication was gastric cancer. The patient was lucky to be confirmed earlier and recovered well after surgery.

For the patients, as most of them lack medical knowledge and out of respect for the elders, they always think the experience of the elders makes sense after the test of time. But the experience may not be suitable for every occasion. Thus if the patient feels sick, he or she should ask for help from doctors. As a doctor, if you find problems, you must communicate with the patient and persuade him or her to get the appropriate examination and treatment. You souldn't be afraid of disputes.

There is also a very classic elder concept, "Break bones for a hundred days". It is believed many people have heard that, that is to say, if you have a bone injury, such as fracture, you need to rest at home for at least 100 days to recover. So is it right? The elders often show the view that when your bones get injured, your Qi gets injured too. It takes a long time to rest well. But how do you see from the modern medical perspective? A patient once had a sprained ankle, and the doctor treated him with a stretch bandage. However, an elder family member advised the patient that he needs one hundred days of lying in bed to recover. He obeyed it for nearly one month and finally formed a deep vein thrombosis of lower limbs and almost died because of pulmonary embolism. Modern medicine has proved that long-term bed rest is a high risk factor of the deep venous thrombosis, which has a most dangerous complication named pulmonary embolism. It means if a patient with broken bones undergoes prolonged bed rest wrongly, he probably dies from the pulmonary embolism with no trouble in the bone. Therefore, the traditional concept of this grandmother phenomenon is worth discussing.

Also, in terms of the "confinement" that women have to go through after giving birth, there are many experiences that have passed down from generation to generation. "Confinement" literally refers to the need of a rest period of about one month after giving birth. This statement originated more than 2,000 years ago from the Western Han Dynasty, when it was called "in the month". Afterwards, it gradually became a process that every mother must have after childbirth. From a scientific point of view, "confinement" is a beneficial transition to help a woman to change from a daughter and wife's role to a mother's role. But some conventional experiences during this time may not have scientific basis. For example, the elders said that a woman who has just given birth could not take a bath during the "confinement" period, because the postpartum Qi and blood are both insufficient. If bathing, they may cause the cold to invade the body, Qi and blood would become stagnant, and irregular menstruation or arthralgia would occur in the future. In the contemporary view, in the old days it was impossible to provide a warm surrounding when taking a bath, so it was very likely to get a cold, while the living conditions nowadays have become much improved and a better environment is available. So women could take a bath during the "confinement" period. Imagine that during the "confinement" period, the mother would have a lot of perspiration, postpartum lochia, and milk secretion, and the skin will become very dirty. If the body is not cleaned for one month, it may not only produce an unpleasant odor, but also weaken the skin, such that pathogens could invade, causing maternal mastitis, folliculitis, endometritis, and so on, and the maternal infection may affect neonatal babies during breastfeeding. Modern research has shown that during the "confinement" period bathing can clean the skin, avoid skin and perineum infection, and help mothers to relieve fatigue and promote sleep. Therefore, it is unscientific to adhere to traditional customs that advise against taking a bath during the "confinement" period. There is also an old folk saying that during the "confinement" period, the mother cannot wash and comb her hair, otherwise she would have a headache in the future. The elders believe that the post-partum women are so weak that washing hair would bring humidity and cold to her head, so it's easy to leave the cause of headache in the future. According to the modern concept, women sweat a lot during delivery and the month after birth. If they do not wash hair for one month, the hair and scalp will become dirty and smelly, even prone to infections. Thus washing hair properly can not only clean scalp and hair roots, but also promote blood circulation in the head, strengthen the hair, avoid hair loss and breakage, and relieve mothers' mood. According to traditional customs it was also not recommended to brush teeth during the "confinement". The elders believe that brushing teeth during the month would hurt the teeth and roots and cause teeth to be loosened and falling off. In the modern view, after eating there may be food residues left in the mouth and the gaps between the teeth. If not brushing teeth for a long time, bacteria may ferment and acidify the residues, causing teeth decalcification, caries or periodontal disease, and also bad breath, mouth ulcers, and so on, and eventually the teeth would be loosening and falling off. Therefore, the view of not brushing teeth not only hardly has scientific reasons, but also may cause a series of problems in your mouth and teeth, such as the loss of teeth. So it is needed to change the views into modern concepts.

For the newborn, the older generation mostly spreads a saying that it is to "squeeze the nipples" for them. In the elders' concept, the nipples will become "Hypoplastic nipples" without squeezing. Especially in the female babies, "Hypoplastic nipples" will make it impossible to feed babies in the future. Many young mothers with inexperience agree to do that, leading to many tragedies.

"Hypoplastic nipples" means the nipples retract medically; it happens not because the mothers don't "squeeze the nipples" of the babies after birth, but because they get congenital diseases such as smooth muscle dysplasia and so on. Pubescent girls have the same problems as they wear bras inaccurately. It is a very dangerous job to "squeeze the nipples" of babies. Some people try their hardest to squeeze out the nipples, which hurt the babies' soft breast skin and then cause skin inflammation and even sepsis. Such examples in life are all around. It can be seen that the "squeezing the nipples" for newborns not only has no scientific basis, but also may bring serious complications such as neonatal infections. It is a wrong traditional concept of the older generation and we need to correct the view.

Currently there are also some traditional concepts of life that do not necessarily contribute to health. For example, most parents taught us to "sit like a bell, stand like a pine", such as sitting on a chair the back must be straight. However, this too stiff sitting posture would cause the back to bear extra pressure and result in lower limbs pain. A doctor from Scotland suggests that it's better for the white-collar workers to sit naturally rather than sitting straight, otherwise the excessive stress on the spine and ligaments is likely to make you feel painful. In the sitting position, the optimal angle between the upper body and the thigh is not a right angle that people usually think, but an elevation angle of 135 degrees. For another example, there is a saying that "A white cover three ugly". So the people of the country, especially women, prefer the fair skin in particular. In the summer, the sun protection measures are quite in place. The legendary 3S — the Slip is kit shirt, the Slop is coated with sunscreen, the Slap is wearing a hat — perhaps can help you to keep skin white and tender, to prevent sunburn and skin cancer, while it is very likely to make your body lack vitamin D. Vitamin D's function includes to strengthen bones, lower fracture risk, reduce bone and joint pain, and relieve muscle weakness, at the same time regulating calcium levels automatically. You should not stay away from the sun completely. What you should do is to find a balance between preventing sunburn and avoiding vitamin D deficiency. For example, try not to go out in the afternoon and try to go out in the morning or evening and so on.

"Dr. Grandma" is a very common phenomenon in our society. Many elders held the view that their life experience is much richer than that of the youngers as they have lived for decades, and they always like to pass on their experience to the younger generation and even interfere in the treatment of diseases. For these "Dr. grandmas", we must show our respect first because they are older, and their life experiences are very helpful and beneficial. Respecting the elders is a virtue in China. Mencius said that you "Expand the respect of the aged in one's family to that of other families; expand the love of the young ones in one's family to that of other families". Zhuangzi said that you "Carry Mount Tai beyond the Beihai Sea is not to do nothing; break branches for the elderly is neither to do nor to do nothing". David Deker said that "Respect for the elderly is natural and normal. Respect is not only expressed verbally, but also in reality". Of course, we should show the most basic respect and courtesy to the elders; but when faced with some unenlightened, obsolete, and even wrong views, we should also point them out. However, we need to pay attention to some details, so that we may not need to directly tell the elderly that the concept is wrong for their dignity. We should show the view in a sincere manner and scientific way, explain why their views are old and wrong, what are the reasons for the mistake, which are the correct practices, and what are the correct reasons, and strive to make "Dr. grandma" convinced. Surely, we should also do extensive education and popularization work in public places and in the media, to inform the public which traditional concepts are correct and which are incorrect and why. Persuade the public to not adopt traditional and unscientific concepts blindly, and meanwhile do not hurt Dr. Grandma's love.

Part III

Medical Communication for Specific Populations

Chapter 6

Health Education, Health Promotion, and Health Management

With the practice of human health, people's understanding of health is becoming more and more comprehensive. The influencing factors of health have also expanded from simple individual factors to cultural and social categories. In 1948, the World Health Organization (WHO) proposed the definition of health as: "Health is a sound state of physical, mental, and social adaptation, not just the absence of disease and infirmity." This definition extended the explanation of health from "biological person without disease" to "social person", linking social interaction, cultural customs, interpersonal relationship with health, and emphasizing the impact of society, culture, politics, and economy on health.[1] In 1978, the WHO reiterated in the Almaty Declaration that "health is not only the absence of disease and suffering, but also a state of perfection in all aspects of physical, mental and social functions." In 1986, the WHO emphasized in the Ottawa Charter that "health should be regarded as a resource of daily life, not a goal of life. Health is a positive concept. It is not only an embodiment of personal physical fitness, but also the resources of society and individuals. In order to achieve a perfect state of physical and mental health and a better fit for society, everyone must have the

---

[1] Fu, H., Zheng, F., & Shi, H. (2011). *Health promotion theory and practice*. Shanghai: Fudan University Press.

ability to recognize and realize these desires, and strive to meet the needs and improve the environment." In 1989, the WHO further improved the concept of health, "health is a good state of physiological, psychological, social adaptation and morality."

The traditional concept of health is "disease-free is health". Modern people's concept of health is overall health. The concept of modern people's health content includes: physical health, mental health, spiritual health, social health, intellectual health, moral health, environmental health, and so on. From the development of the definition of health, we can see that health is both a multi-dimensional good state and an important resource. Resources need to be managed, through which they can be maximized.

1. Health education, health promotion, and health management

For a long time in the past, people's understanding of health education was still limited to health propaganda. But health propaganda is not the same as health education. Health propaganda refers to the untargeted one-way communication process of information such as health knowledge and health policies. Instead of focusing on feedback and effects, the process aims to increase the accumulation of people's health knowledge. However, empirical evidence shows that the accumulation of knowledge cannot effectively achieve the effect of behavioral transformation, so the effect of health propaganda is often unsatisfactory.

Health education in China has developed from health propaganda. Today, the connotation and methods of health education have surpassed health propaganda. The World Health Organization defines health education as: "To help and encourage people to have the desire to be healthy, and to guide how to achieve such a goal; each person tries to do his or her own or collective best; and to guide people to seek appropriate help when necessary". Combined with the definition and practical experience of the WHO, the modern definition of health education in our country refers to "through planned, organized, and systematic social education activities, people can consciously adopt healthy behaviors and lifestyles, eliminate or mitigate risk factors affecting health, prevent diseases, promote health, improve quality of life, and evaluate the effect of education". The core of health education is to educate people to establish health awareness, to promote people to change unhealthy behaviors and lifestyles, to develop a good behavior and lifestyle, in order to reduce or eliminate the risk factors affecting health. Health education can help people understand which behaviors affect health, and consciously choose healthy behaviors and lifestyles. The purpose of health education includes: to enhance people's health and enable individuals and groups to achieve the goal of health; to improve and maintain health; to prevent the occurrence of abnormal deaths, diseases, and disabilities; to improve interpersonal relationships and enhance people's ability of self-health care, to get rid of superstitions, abandon bad habits, develop good health habits, advocate a civilized, healthy, and scientific lifestyle; to enhance the concept of health so as to understand, support, and advocate health policies and healthy environments. In short, health education is to promote people to adopt a healthy lifestyle, which can achieve physical and psychological health, and reduce the morbidity, disability rate, and mortality of diseases.

The significance of health education is to raise people's awareness of health, so that they can understand some basic health care knowledge (basic content and implementation methods) and develop scientific, civilized and healthy living habits. Health education can be carried out in various ways and should be popularized to every member of society. However, since society is composed of members of different structures, with different ages, genders, levels, and needs, health education must be carried out in accordance with different learning needs and starting points of different groups, and different educational methods and contents should be designed. It is necessary to carry out targeted skills training and learning, such as family nursing, infant care, emergency rescue, and other scientific knowledge, but also to carry out pure self-improvement, learning activities of cultivate health, such as aerobics, calligraphy and painting, flower cultivation, reading, and learning. In many cases, learning for the joy is also the purpose of motivating people to read. The goal of health education is to carry out various forms of health education activities, popularize health knowledge, enhance people's health awareness and self-care ability, and improve the health literacy of the whole people, based on the community and focusing on major health issues, key places, and key populations.

As mentioned above, the core of health education is to promote individuals or groups to establish health awareness and change unhealthy behaviors and lifestyles, especially to change organizational behaviors. However, according to the practical experience of health education in many countries in the world, behavioral change is a long-term and complex process, which depends not only on subjective wishes of individual, but also on supportive health policies, environment, and health services and other related factors. Under such circumstances, health promotion begins to develop rapidly.

Health promotion was first put forward by the World Health Organization at the first International Health Promotion Conference in Ottawa, Canada on November 21, 1986. It refers to the use of administrative or organizational means to broadly coordinate the society. All relevant departments, as well as communities, families, and individuals, fulfill their respective responsibilities for health and jointly maintain and promote a social behavior and social strategy for health. The Ottawa Charter, issued by the conference, states that "Health promotion is the process of motivating people to enhance, maintain and improve their own health". Brundtland, the former Director-General of the World Health Organization, made a clearer explanation of health promotion at the Fifth Global Conference on Health Promotion in 2000: "Health promotion is to make people do everything possible to keep their spirits and bodies in the best state. And its aim is to make people know how to stay healthy, to keep healthy lifestyle, and to make healthy choices." According to the latest statement in the *American Journal of Health Promotion*, "Health promotion is the science (and art) that help people change their lifestyles to achieve optimal health. Optimal health is defined as the level of physical, emotional, social, mental and intellectual health. Lifestyle changes are facilitated by the combination of cognitive improvement, behavioral change and the creation of supportive environments. Among the three, the supportive environment is the biggest contributor to sustained improvement of health." In the contemporary concept of health promotion, people's awareness of empowerment is especially prominent, and they improve their health through the promotion of power and ability. In terms

Table 6.1 Relationships and differences between health publicity, health education, and health promotion.

	Health propaganda	Health education	Health promotion
Connotation	Information + propaganda	Knowledge + belief + behavior change	Health education + policy environment support
Methods	Mass communication	Combining communication with education, focusing on education	Health education + social mobilization + creating an environment
Characteristics	One-way propaganda	Taking behavior change as the core	Full social participation, multi-sectoral cooperation, comprehensive intervention on risk factors affecting health
Effect	Accumulation of health knowledge	Changes in knowledge, beliefs, and behaviors can bring about improvement of individual and group health level	Improvement of individual and group health level, creation of healthy environment, effect from persistence

of affiliation, health promotion includes health education, while health education includes health propaganda (see Table 6.1).[2]

In the Ottawa Charter, WHO proposes five strategies for health promotion, including: formulating public policies for health; creating a supportive environment; strengthening community action; developing personal skills; adjusting the direction of health services.

(1) To formulate public policies for health. Health promotion goes beyond health care. It puts health issues on the agenda of all departments and leaders at all levels, so that they can understand the impact of their decisions on health consequences and take responsibility for health.

Health promotion policies are a combination of diverse and complementary aspects, including legislation, fiscal measures, taxation,

---

[2] Wei, Q., & Mi, G. (2005). *Community health education and health promotion.* Beijing: Chemical Industry Press.

and organizational change. This coordinated action has brought about greater equality in health, income, and social policies. The joint action aims to ensure safer and healthier supply of goods and services, healthier public services and a cleaner and more pleasant environment.

Health promotion policies need to identify barriers to the adoption of health public policies in non-health sectors and ways to overcome them. The target must be to make it easier for decision-makers to make healthier choices.

(2) To create a supportive environment. Our society is complex and interconnected. Health cannot be separated from other goals. Human beings are inextricably linked to their living environment, which is the basis for a socio-ecological approach to health. The general guiding principle is the same for the world, countries, regions and communities, that is, the need to promote mutual preservation — our communities and natural environment need to protect each other. It should be emphasized that the protection of the world's natural resources is a global responsibility.

Changes in lifestyle, work and leisure patterns have important implications for health. Work and leisure should be healthy resources for people, and the work of social organizations should help create a healthy society. Health promotion is to create a safe, comfortable, satisfying, and pleasant life and working conditions.

A systematic assessment of the impact of rapid environmental changes on health, especially in areas of technology, work, energy production, and urbanization, is essential and must be promoted through health promotion activities to ensure a positive impact on public health. Any health promotion strategy must be put forward to protect nature, create a good environment, and protect natural resources.

(3) To strengthen community action. Health promotion is to achieve healthier goals through concrete and effective community actions, including prioritization, decision-making, design of strategies and implementation. The core issue in this process is to empower the communities to be masters of their own lives and participate actively and dominate their own destiny.

Community development relies on the use of existing human and material resources in the community to enhance self-help and social support and to form a flexible system to promote public participation in health work and to guide the development of health work. This requires full and continuous access to health information and learning opportunity as well as financial support.

(4) To develop personal skills. Health promotion supports the development of individual and social development through the provision of information, health education, and improved life skills. The purpose of this is to enable the masses to more effectively maintain their own health and the environment in which they live and make healthy choices. It is extremely important to promote the lifelong learning of the masses, to understand the various stages of life and to deal with chronic diseases and injuries. Schools, families, workplaces, and communities have a responsibility to do so. Such activities need to be done through educational, professional, commercial, and volunteer groups and within these institutions.

(5) To adjust the direction of health services. The responsibility of health promotion in health services is shared by individuals, community organizations, health professionals, health services, and the government. They must work together in the health care system to meet health needs.

The role of the health sector is not only to provide clinical and therapeutic services, but also to adhere to the direction of health promotion. Health services need to expand the power of appointment to enhance empowerment, which is accepted and respects cultural needs. The power of appointment supports the needs of individuals and communities for a healthier life and opens channels between the health sector and the wider social, political, economic, and physical environment sectors. Adjusting the direction of health services also requires more emphasis on the transformation of health research and professional education and training. This requires changes in the attitude and organizations of health services, based on the total needs of a complete person.

The Ottawa Charter also proposes three basic strategies for health promotion:

(1) To advocate: Advocate government departments, the whole society and individuals to pay attention to health, advocate health support

policies, advocate health support environment and convenience measures, and advocate the willingness of individuals to make healthy behavior changes. Good health is a major resource for social, economic, and personal development and an important part of the quality of life. Political, economic, social, cultural, environmental, behavioral, and biological factors all contribute to health or damage it. The aim of the health promotion initiative is to make these factors beneficial to health through support for health.

(2) To empower: Helping government departments, social units, and individuals to equip them with appropriate capabilities, such as knowledge, skills, decision-making judgment and action, to maximize the influence and control of various factors related to a region or individual's own health, and to be able to take responsibility of the implementation of a health promotion project. Health promotion focuses on achieving equality in health. The goal of the health promotion initiative is to narrow the gap between current health conditions and to ensure equal opportunities and resources to enable all people to realize their full potential for health, including the solid foundations, knowledge, life skills, and opportunities to support the environment when choosing health measures. Unless people have the potential to control these conditions that determine health, they cannot reach their fullest health potential. In this regard, men and women should enjoy equal rights.

(3) To coordinate: Coordinate the relevant interests and actions of the government, society and individuals in health promotion, and form a cooperative and mutually beneficial health promotion work system or alliance. The necessary conditions and prospects for health cannot be solely committed by the health sector. More importantly, health promotion requires the coordination of the actions of all relevant sectors: government, health and other socio-economic sectors, nongovernmental and volunteer organizations, regional administrations, industrial and mining enterprises, and the media sector. People from all walks of life participate as individuals, families, and communities. The primary responsibility of all professional and social groups as well as health personnel is to coordinate the participation of different sectors of society in health.

There are differences and connections between health education and health promotion.

Firstly, health education requires people to consciously adopt healthy behaviors and lifestyles through changes in their own cognitions, attitudes, values, and skills. Therefore, in principle, health education is most applicable to people who can change their behavior by changing their own factors. While health promotion provides a supportive environment in terms of organization, policy, economy, and law, which is supportive or restrictive to behavior change. In other words, health promotion provides a supportive environment for health education.

Secondly, health education is the core of health promotion. Health promotion needs the promotion and implementation of health education to create an atmosphere of health promotion. Without health education, health promotion lacks a foundation. Health education must be supported by the environment and policies to develop itself toward health promotion step by step, otherwise its function will be greatly limited. Compared with health education, health promotion integrates objective support and subjective participation. Health promotion includes health education, which is the change of knowledge, beliefs, and behaviors of individuals and groups, and environmental support.

We have to admit, health education is the foundation and the guide of health promotion. Health education plays an important role in promoting behavior change. It also plays an important role in the process of stimulating leaders' political will to develop health promotion, promoting the willingness to support the social system, promoting the willingness of the masses to participate actively, and promoting health promotion atmosphere. At the same time, the support of government's commitments, policies, regulations, organizations, and environment, which are included in health promotion, is a strong support for health education. Without health promotion, the necessary conditions for changing behavior provided by health education, such as community development, social mobilization, cultural cultivation, resource input, and so on, will be inevitably weakened or absent. When the target public make healthy behavior choices and changes, they will not be able to do so because of inadequate support.

Besides, health management is also crucial. Management refers to the activity process in which the managers in a certain organization coordinate the activities of others through the implementation of planning, organization, leadership, coordination, control, and other functions, so that others can achieve their established goals together with themselves. It is the most common and important activity in various human activities. Health management is to apply the concept of management to the field of health maintenance and health promotion, and plan, organize, direct, coordinate and control health resources, improve health, and achieve maximum health benefits. Health management refers to the process of comprehensive management of health risk factors of individuals or groups. Its purpose is to mobilize the initiative of individuals and groups, and effectively use limited resources to achieve maximum health effects.

The concept of health management was proposed firstly in the United States in the late 1950s. Its core content is that medical insurance institutions can effectively control the occurrence or development of diseases by carrying out systematic health management for their medical insurance customers (including patients with diseases or high-risk groups), significantly reduce the probability of accidents and actual medical expenses, thereby reducing the loss of medical insurance claims. The original concept of Managed Care in the United States also included the most cost-effective prescription agreement between medical insurance institutions and medical institutions to ensure lower medical costs for health insurance customers, thereby reducing the reimbursement burden on medical insurance companies.

In a relatively narrow sense, health management refers to the establishment of exclusive health records based on the results of health examination, the evaluation of health status, and a targeted personalized health management scheme (prescription), according to which, one-to-one consulting guidance and tracking counseling service are provided by professionals to enable customers to obtain comprehensive health maintenance and support services from social, psychological, environmental, nutritional, sports, and other angles.

Health management has developed for decades in Europe and the United States. At present, scholars in Europe and the United States have expressed the concept of health management as: "Health management refers to an activity process that comprehensively detects, evaluates and effectively intervenes the health risk factors of individuals or groups.

Its main purpose is to achieve maximum health improvement effect by improving or changing the means and product delivery of health services as well as improving the effective organizational behavior of public health with minimum input. Health management is to provide a scientific and healthy lifestyle to health demanders, change passive health care to active health management, and protect and promote human health more effectively."

In China, the idea of health management was first proposed by Mr. Su Taiyang in the journal of *Health Medicine* when he was the editor-in-chief. "Health management is to use the theory and methods of management science, through purposeful, planned, and organized management, to mobilize the enthusiasm of all organizations and members of the whole society, and to intervene effectively in the health of groups and individuals, so as to achieve the purpose of maintaining, consolidating, promoting group and individual health." In another health management textbook edited by Chen Junshi and Huang Jianshi, health management is defined as: "Health management is to monitor, analyze and evaluate the health of individuals or groups, to provide health consultation and guidance, and to intervene health risk factors. The purpose of health management is to mobilize the initiative of individuals and groups as well as the whole society, and effectively use limited resources to achieve maximum health effects. The specific approach of health management for individuals and groups (including the government) is to provide targeted scientific health information and to create conditions for action to improve health." It is the most widely cited concept of health management in China.

Health management has the following main characteristics:

(1) The core is to control the risk factors of health. Health risk factors include variable risk factors and immutable risk factors. Unhealthy lifestyles, such as unreasonable diets, lack of exercise, smoking, and alcoholism, are risk factors that can be controlled through self-behavior changes and belong to variable risk factors. Others, such as age, gender, and family history of disease, are not risk factors that can be changed through self-behavior, but are immutable risk factors.

(2) Health management is a combination of primary, secondary, and tertiary prevention. Primary prevention, also known as etiological

prevention, is to take measures for the cause or risk factors before the disease (or injury) occurs, reduce the level of harmful exposure, and enhance the individual's ability to resist harmful exposure to prevent the occurrence of the disease (or injury) or at least delay the occurrence of disease (or injury). For example, in people with a family history of diabetes, we recommend that they take measures to control their weight, control their diet, strengthen exercise, and slow down the occurrence of diabetes, which belongs to the primary prevention. Secondary prevention, that is, early detection and early treatment of disease, also known as preclinical prevention (or pre-symptomatic prevention), that is, "three early" preventive measures for early detection, early diagnosis, and early treatment in the preclinical stage of the disease. This level of prevention is through early detection, early diagnosis, and appropriate treatment to prevent changes in the preclinical or early clinical stage of the disease, can make the disease to be detected and treated at an early stage, to avoid or reduce complications, sequelae, and disability, or to shorten the time of disability. For example, in obesity and people with family history of diabetes, we regularly do screening for diabetes in order to find early detection of diabetes, which is secondary prevention. Tertiary prevention, namely, treatment and prevention of disability, also known as clinical prevention. Tertiary prevention can prevent disability and promote functional recovery, improve quality of life, prolong life, and reduce mortality. For example, in patients with diabetes, we give active hypoglycemic therapy and other adjuvant treatments and control blood sugar in the target range, in order to delay the occurrence of diabetic complications, which is tertiary prevention.

(3) The service process of health management is a circular running cycle. The implementation of health management includes health monitoring (collecting personal health information of service object, which is the premise and basis for continuous implementation of health management), health assessment (predicting the risk of various diseases, which is the fundamental guarantee for implementing health management), and health interventions (helping service object to take action to control risk factors, which is the ultimate goal of implementing health management). Through these three links, the entire

service process is continuously cycled to reduce or lower the number and level of risk factors and maintain a low level of risk. For example, for a middle-aged male with obesity, first collect all his personal health information, including diet, exercise, work, lifestyle, and some basic health examination data (such as blood sugar, blood pressure, etc.), and then assess the risk of his various diseases (such as diabetes, hypertension, cardiovascular and cerebrovascular diseases, etc.), and finally help him to make changes in some bad lifestyle choices and behavior, in order to delay the occurrence of disease and achieve the goal of health management. Thus, it is a cycle process of health management.

The contents of health management mainly include:

(1) Collecting health-related information. Systematically and comprehensively collecting health-related information of individuals or groups is the basis for health assessment. Health-related information mainly includes basic personal information (gender, age, sex, race, etc.) and past medical history (with or without chronic history such as diabetes, hypertension, history of cancer, history of surgery, etc.) and family history of disease (family history of cancer, family history of cardiovascular and cerebrovascular diseases, etc.), current disease and health status, general physical examination (height, weight, waist circumference, blood pressure, etc.), auxiliary examination (blood routine, urine routine, blood sugar, blood lipids and electrocardiogram, B-mode ultrasonography, chest radiograph, etc.) and lifestyle (diet, exercise, smoking, drinking, sleep, etc.), and so on, can also increase other special contents according to the actual situation of individuals or groups.

(2) Conduct a health assessment. Based on the collected health information, the health risk factors of individuals or groups and the risk of morbidity or death in the future are assessed by epidemiological and health statistics methods. In the assessment of disease and death, a prediction and assessment model is usually formed on the basis of a large sample population research, and the health information of individuals or groups is substituted or compared to assess the risk

of disease incidence or death of individuals or groups in the future. However, such models are constantly adjusted and improved with changes in research methods, techniques, and population-related factors. In the assessment of health risk factors, the main and changeable health risk factors for chronic diseases according to the degree of harm of different factors are determined according to the harm degree of different factors and the intensity of association with the diseases, so as to carry out targeted intervention and management in the future.

(3) Implementing health interventions. Health interventions are the core of health management. Based on the results of the health assessment, develop health management plan and discuss with the clients to determine the goal of the health intervention, the health risk factors of priority intervention, and reasonable and feasible intervention measures. Interventions in health management are more individualized than health education and health promotion. With the active participation of the clients, the clients are assisted in taking actions in various forms to correct unhealthy lifestyles and behavioral habits, to control, reduce, eliminate health risk factors, and achieve the goal of the health management plan. After the implementation of health intervention for a certain period of time, health information can be collected for health assessment again, so as to evaluate the effectiveness of intervention measures and to improve and adjust health intervention plans and measures.

From the content of health management, it can be seen that health management is a cycle-by-cycle process. Long-term, systematic health management can maintain and promote the health of individuals or groups.

The basic strategy of health management, from the macro perspective, is to make suggestions for the health resource management of the whole nation at the national level, to make evidence-based health management decisions by providing accurate health monitoring information, and to scientifically adjust the overall strategic layout of national medical treatment and health and make contributions to improving the health level of the whole nation. From the micro perspective, it includes six forms: lifestyle management, demand management, disease management, disaster injury management, disability management, and integrated population health management.

Health education, health promotion, and health management all take the collection of baseline data — assessment — intervention — effect evaluation as the main line in the analysis and solution of problems. But health management introduces the concept of health risk assessment and management. In the pre-planning research assessment, health education focuses more on knowledge, attitude, belief, behavior, and other aspects. Health management also places emphasis on physical examination data and emphasizes long-term and continuous management of lifestyle and behavior. In the process of planning, health education pays more attention to the change of knowledge, attitude, and behaviors of target public. Health management should propose individualized intervention measures based on the results of risk assessment. In the process of implementing intervention, health education often uses strategies such as education, environment, and policy. The main means of intervention are education and management. Health education is a very basic and important method and strategy for both individual and group health management. When evaluating the effect of intervention, health education is divided into process evaluation, effect evaluation, and outcome evaluation, which are similar in health management. However, health management focuses more on behavioral changes, improvement of health indicators, and changes in health risks.

2. Healthy behavior model

Healthy behavior refers to habitual behavior that is beneficial to health. In the practice of health education and promotion, researchers gradually explored model of individual health behaviors, which can be used to explain the formation and influencing factors of health behaviors. Commonly used models include the KABP model, the health belief model, the planned behavior theory, and the behavioral change model and the change stage.

2.1. *The KABP model*

In the model of knowledge, attitude, belief, and practice (KABP or KAP), in health education and health promotion, "K" is knowledge, "A" is attitude, and "P" is practice. It is the most commonly used model to explain how individual knowledge and beliefs affect changes in healthy behavior, which was put forward by Coaster and Briton in the 1960s. The theory divides the change of human behavior into three successive processes: Knowledge, Attitude, and Practice. Among them, "knowledge" is the knowing and understanding of relevant knowledge, which is the basis; "attitude" is the correct belief and positive attitude, which is the driving force; "practice" is the action, which is the process of promoting health behavior and eliminating harmful behaviors and the goal. When people understand the relevant health knowledge and establish positive and correct beliefs and attitude, it is possible to actively form health-friendly behaviors and change health-threatening behaviors. The transformation from knowledge to behavior requires external conditions. Health education is an important external condition that promotes the transformation of knowledge into behavior.

For example, smoking is a health-threatening behavior. The following steps are usually required to change this harmful behavior through the "KAP" model and finally let the smoker reach the goal of quitting smoking. First of all, it is necessary to make smokers understand the harmful components of tobacco, the health hazards of smoking, the benefits of quitting smoking, and how to quit smoking, which is the basis for smokers to quit. Secondly, let smokers establish the belief that smoking is harmful to health and that they can successfully quit smoking through efforts, so that smokers have the motivation to implement the action of quitting smoking. Of course, the ultimate transformation from knowledge to behavior is a long and complex process, which is influenced by many factors. Knowledge is a necessary but not sufficient condition for behavior change. The process from knowledge to behavior is generally as follows: information communication → awareness of information → arousing interest → feeling needed → thinking seriously → believing in information → generating motivation → trying to behave resolutely → dynamic stereotype → behavioral establishment. There are two main key steps: the establishment of beliefs and the change of attitude. There is no causal relationship between knowledge, attitude, and practice, but it must be inevitable. After the attitude is established, if there is no prerequisite for resolute change of attitude, the goal of achieving behavioral change will still lead to failure. In the practice of health education, there are often cases of "knowing but not believing" and "believing but not doing". "Knowing and not believing" may be due to the credibility, infectiveness, and authority of the disseminated information are not strong enough to stimulate people's beliefs. For example, for smokers, smoking is harmful to health. If the communicator is a smoker, then the reliability of his/her communication of knowledge is worthy of being confused. Then the effect of education and communication cannot be achieved. "believing but not doing" may be due to some insurmountable obstacles in people's behavioral establishing or changing, or a large cost needed to pay, which offset the benefits of behavior. So, no action is produced. For example, the smoker knows that smoking has many hazards, but since he has been smoking for many years, it has become a habit in his life. And because his job is in sales, he often needs to hand over tobacco and toast and it is hard to quit, which forms an obstacle to his smoking cessation. At this point, if he learns that his close friend of his similar age, because of long-term smoking, is suffering from lung cancer, it is likely to prompt him to finally make up his mind to quit smoking. Therefore, only by comprehensively mastering the complex process of the transformation of knowledge, attitude, and practice, can the adverse effects be eliminated or weakened in a timely and effective manner and the enabling environment be formed, so as to achieve the purpose of changing behavior.

2.2. *Health belief model*

The health belief model (HBM) is a health education model that changes people's behaviors by interfering with people's perceptions, attitudes, beliefs, and other psychological activities. It was born in the early 1950s and is one of the most widely used theoretical frameworks in health behavior research.

Social psychologists in the 1950s explained the reasons for the widespread failure of people to participate in the prevention and detection of diseases from a psychosocial perspective. For example, in the case of pulmonary tuberculosis detected by X-rays, Hochbaum (1958) found that 82% of those in the group who believed in the susceptibility of tuberculosis and the benefits of early detection had at least one X-ray examination during the investigation, while 64% of those who believed in susceptibility but did not believe in the benefits of early detection were willing to do X-ray fluoroscopy. On the contrary, only 29% of those who had only beneficial beliefs but no susceptibility beliefs were willing to take X-ray examination; if neither belief existed, only 21% of them had X-ray examination during the investigation.

Subsequent researchers continued to generalize the perceptions of obstacles, behavioral cues, and self-efficacy, and finally formed a complete health belief model (Figure 6.1).

The health belief model is a theoretical model to explain health-related behaviors by using social psychology, which emphasizes the importance of perception in decision-making. Many factors can affect perception. The theory holds that belief is the basis for people to adopt healthy behaviors. If people have beliefs about diseases and health, they will adopt healthy behaviors and change risky behaviors. When people think about whether to adopt a healthy behavior, they first judge the threat of the disease, then judge the value of preventing the disease, the expectation of adopting healthy behavior to improve the health condition and the ability to overcome obstacles to action, and finally decide whether to adopt the healthy behavior.

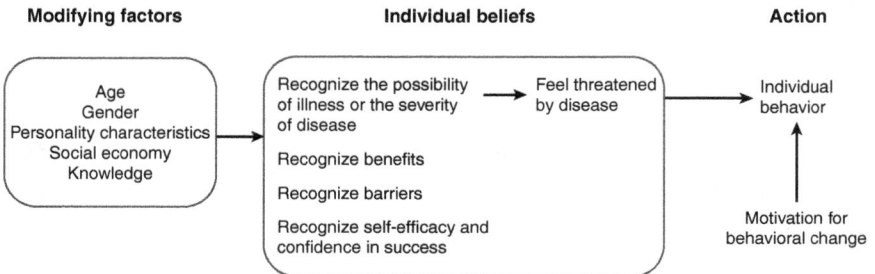

Modifying factors	Individual beliefs	Action

| Age
Gender
Personality characteristics
Social economy
Knowledge | Recognize the possibility of illness or the severity of disease → Feel threatened by disease

Recognize benefits

Recognize barriers

Recognize self-efficacy and confidence in success | Individual behavior

↑

Motivation for behavioral change |

Figure 6.1   Health belief model.

(1) Perceived threat

The threat of disease that people perceive, includes the perceived suscepti-bility of the disease and the perceived severity of the disease. If an indi-vidual believes that the more serious the disease, the more likely he or she is to suffer from a disease, the more likely he or she is to take action.

(2) Perceived benefit and barrier

That is, the subjective judgment of the individual on the benefits and bar-riers brought about by the adoption or abandonment of certain behaviors, namely the general perception of advantages and disadvantages. The greater the perceived benefits and the smaller the barriers, the easier it is to adopt or abandon the behavior.

(3) Self-efficacy

That is, the judgment and evaluation of an individual's ability to adopt or abandon a certain behavior, which is similar to self-confidence. This con-cept derives from Bandura's social cognitive theory (Bandura, 1997). Even if an individual perceives the seriousness of the problem, he or she has insufficient belief in his or her own ability to form a belief in change.

(4) Cues to action

This is the "final driving force" that leads to changes in individual behavior, such as physical discomfort, media reports about the serious consequences of the behavior, or advice from doctors or family members, and so on.

For example, a young man recently finds that he suffers from diabetes during a routine physical examination. Because of his obesity, doctors recommend him to lose weight and increase exercise, and take at least 30 minutes' moderate-intensity physical activity every day. He realizes that his diabetes is associated with obesity (perceived susceptibility) and diabetes could lead to acute complications such as ketoacidosis, hypergly-cemia and hyperosmotic syndrome, hypoglycemia coma, and may lead to chronic complications such as cardiovascular and cerebrovascular dis-eases, and disease of kidneys, ocular and peripheral neuropathy, causing organ dysfunction and disability (perceived severity). Under the doctor's education, he realizes that losing weight and increasing exercise are good for controlling diabetes (perceived behavioral benefit). At the same time, he also feels that losing weight is too difficult for him from being obese to being normal type (perceived behavioral barrier). But he believes that through his own unremitting efforts, he can gradually increase exercise and lose weight (self-efficacy). One of his good friends has recently suffered from an acute myocardial infarction due to diabetes and was sent to the hospital. This is very motivating to him (cues to action). Combining all these factors, the young man finally starts his weight loss and exercise program. This is an example of health belief model.

2.3. *Self-efficacy theory*

In 1977, American psychologist Bandura proposed the Self-Efficacy Theory from the perspective of social learning. Self-efficacy refers to the effectiveness or validity of an individual in dealing with internal and external environmental events. It also refers to the subjective judgment of the individual's ability to organize, execute a specific behavior, and achieve the expected results, that is, the individual's self-confidence and self-control ability to successfully adopt the healthy behavior and achieve the desired results due to his or her ability to control the internal and external factors.

The function of self-efficacy is mainly to regulate and control behavior and influence behavioral results through behavioral regulation. Self-efficacy regulates behavior mainly in the following aspects:

(1) To affect people's choice and persistence of behavior. People with a high sense of self-efficacy tend to choose tasks which are suitable for their ability level and challenging, while those with a low sense of self-efficacy tend to choose the opposite.

(2) To affect people's efforts and attitudes toward difficulties. People with a high sense of self-efficacy are more confident and brave to face difficulties and challenges, They believe that they can overcome difficulties through hard work. Therefore, they will strive to pursue and achieve their goals. On the contrary, those with a low sense of self-efficacy will hesitate and be at a loss in the face of difficulties because they doubt their abilities, and even dare not ask about the actions and tasks they can perform.

(3) To affect people's way of thinking and behavioral efficiency. People with low sense of self-efficacy are always worried that they will fail, which affects their actions and the formation of new behaviors and the performance of new behaviors, resulting in low capacity and efficiency of behavior. On the contrary, people with strong sense of self-efficacy focus their attention on actively analyzing and solving problems. They go up to difficulties and pursue persistently. In the face of difficulties, they often make their thinking and problem-solving skills to be extraordinary, showing high-quality behavioral ability and efficiency.

(4) To affect people's attribution. People with high sense of self-efficacy often attribute failure to their lack of effort; while those with low sense of self-efficacy often attribute failure to their lack of ability and talent.

Self-efficacy is the basis of human behavioral motivation, health and individual achievement, which is an important factor in determining whether people can produce behavioral motivation and behavior. Only when people believe that their actions can lead to expected results, are they willing to take action. Otherwise, people will not have strong motivations or long-term persistence in the face of difficulties. People with high sense of self-efficacy are more likely to adopt the recommended health-promoting behavior.

The influencing factors of self-efficacy are influenced by four kinds of information sources. Self-efficacy can be generated and improved through the following four ways:

(1) The direct success experience of the individual. Direct experience, such as behavioral success or failure, comes from personal experience, which has the greatest impact on self-efficacy. Successful experiences can improve the individual's sense of self-efficacy. A success can help people increase their expectations of mastering a certain behavior skillfully, which is the most powerful evidence of their ability to perform the behavior. For example, a diabetic can control his blood sugar well by controlling his diet, losing weight, and

increasing exercise, which will increase his confidence and improve his self-efficacy. He will be convinced that he has the ability to achieve the goal of controlling blood sugar through "holding your mouth and stepping forward".

(2) The indirect success experience of others. Indirect experience is obtained by observing the behavior of others, seeing that others have successfully completed a certain behavior with good results, and enhancing the self-confidence that one can also complete the behavior through efforts and persistence. For example, an obese patient always plans to lose weight, but he never succeeds. One day, he meets his former companion, who used to be obese. Now, he has lost a lot of weight through exercise and healthy diet. Not only has his body become symmetrical, but also his original hypertension has disappeared, which greatly increases the confidence of the obese patient to lose weight and begin to work hard to implement it.

(3) Verbal persuasion. It refers to a way to improve people's self-efficacy and self-confidence in performing certain behaviors by changing people's knowledge and attitude, through persuasive advice, advice, explanation, and guidance. Verbal persuasion is simple and easy to use. However, due to the lack of experience, the self-efficacy that is formed often lacks firmness. For example, doctors often persuade smokers not to smoke, which is very simple and easy to do. But whether this kind of persuasion can improve the smoker's self-efficacy for quitting smoking, or how long it can last even after the formation of self-efficacy for quitting smoking, it is worth discussing.

(4) Cultivate and regulate emotional and physiological states. In his "desensitization" study, Bandura found that psychological state is one of the important factors affecting self-efficacy. Unhealthy emotions such as anxiety, nervousness, and depression can affect people's judgments of their abilities. By eliminating negative emotions and stimulating positive emotions, people can improve their self-confidence in their abilities. For example, a diabetic patient, through diet control and increased exercise, finds that his blood sugar does not obviously improve and still does not meet the standard, so he is very depressed. At this time, his family and doctors always encourage him and firmly believe that he will finally control his blood sugar through

their unremitting efforts. Through the encouragement of the surrounding crowd, the patient regains his confidence, increases his self-efficacy, and firmly believes that he can achieve the goal of controlling blood sugar; then he continues to adhere to diet control and active exercise, and ultimately achieves the goal of blood sugar control.

2.4. *Theory of reasoned action and theory of planned behavior*

In 1967, American scholars Fishbein and Ajzen put forward the theory of reasoned action (TRA), also known as the theory of reasoned behavior, which was mainly used to analyze how attitudes consciously affect individual behaviors and how attitudes are formed based on cognitive information. The basic assumption is that people are rational and combine various information to consider the meaning and consequences of their actions before making a certain behavior. The theory holds that behavioral intention is the most direct factor affecting behavior, and behavioral intention is determined by behavioral attitude and subjective norm. Theory of planned behavior (TPB) was developed by Ajzen based on the theory of reasoned action to introduce perceived behavioral control (Figure 6.2). According to the theory, besides being determined by attitudes and subjective norm, behavioral intention is also influenced by perceived behavioral control. Perceived behavioral control is the degree of perception that an individual controls his or her behavior, which is determined by both control belief and perceived promotion factor. Control beliefs are people's perceptions of their abilities, resources, and opportunities, and perception promotion factors are people's estimation of the importance of these resources.

In these two theories, behavior refers to the target action taken by the individual at a certain time and in a specific context. Behavioral intention is the measure by which the person intends to engage in a particular behavior. Attitude refers to the individual's positive or negative feelings about behavior, determined by the main beliefs about the outcome of the behavior and the estimation of the importance of the outcome. Subjective norms reflect the perception of other people's

Theory of Reasoned Action

Theory of Planned Behavior

Belief in behavior

Judgement of behavioral result

Belief in social norms

Motivation to comply with social norms

Belief in control

Insight

Attitude towards behavior

Subjective behavioral norms

Perceived behavioral control

Behavioral intention

Behavior

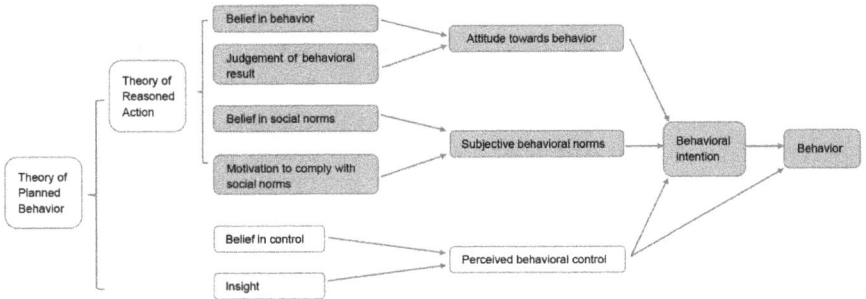

Figure 6.2   Theory of reasoned action and theory of planned behavior.

Note: The shaded part is the theory of reasoned action, which is all displayed as the theory of planned behavior.

evaluation of a certain behavior, which is determined by the degree of individual's trust in what other people think should be done and the level of trust that the individual thinks others should do and the level of motivation that is consistent with others' opinions. Early subjective norms only included how much a certain behavior is permitted in a social community, namely, injunctive norm. However, it is gradually found that the individual's understanding of how others in the group behave can also significantly affect the behavioral intention. So, the descriptive norm is added to the theory. For example, on college campuses in the United States, college students often know that injunctive norms do not recommend excessive drinking. But if they feel that other college students are drinking too much, they are more likely to start drinking themselves. The theory of planned behavior is developed on the basis of the theory of reasoned action. It adds a self-perceived behavioral control, which is a barrier reflecting personal past experience and expectations. The more resources and opportunities individuals think they have, the less expected barriers, the stronger the perceived behavioral control of behaviors. There are two ways of its influence. One is to have motivational implications for behavioral intention; the other is to directly predict behavior. For example, to intervene smokers with the theory of planned behavior, so as to influence their intention to smoke and change their smoking behavior. In view of behavioral attitude toward smoking, the hazards of smoking can be vigorously publicized on various occasions. For subjective norms, smoking cessation lectures can be held to continuously strengthen the communication of correct knowledge of smoking control. For perceived behavioral control, anti-smoking rules and regulations can be formulated in the community, and the staff should discourage people who smoke in public, impose fines when necessary, and restrict their smoking behavior in public places, so as to let them perceive the obstacles of smoking.

The theory of planned behavior has the following main points:

(1) The behavior under complete control of non-personal will is not only affected by behavioral intention, but also restricted by the actual control conditions such as individual ability, opportunity, and resources of the execution behavior. Under the condition of sufficient actual control conditions, the behavioral intention directly determines the behavior.

(2) Accurate perceived behavioral control reflects the actual control conditions, so it can be used as an alternative measurement indicator of actual control conditions, directly predicting the possibility of behavior occurrence, and the accuracy of prediction depends on the true degree of perceived behavioral control.

(3) Behavioral attitude, subjective norms, and perceived behavioral control are the three main variables that determine behavioral intention. The more positive attitude, the greater the support of significant others, the stronger the perceived behavioral control, the greater the behavioral intention and vice versa.

(4) Individuals have a large number of beliefs about behavior, but only a relatively small number of behavioral beliefs can be acquired at a specific time and environment. These acquired beliefs are also called prominent beliefs, which are the cognitive and emotional basis of behavioral attitude, subjective norms, and perceived behavioral control.

(5) Individual and sociocultural factors (such as personality, intelligence, experience, age, gender, cultural background, etc.) indirectly affect behavioral attitude, subjective norms and perceived behavioral control by influencing behavioral beliefs, and ultimately affect behavioral intention and behaviors.

(6) Behavioral attitude, subjective norms, and perceived behavioral control can be conceptually completely distinguished, but sometimes they may share a common belief base, so they are both independent and interrelated.

Although the theory of reasoned action and the theory of planned behavior are highly praised by many researchers for their simplicity and validity of prediction, they do not fully consider the influence of environmental factors on people's behavior. Consequently, subsequent researchers added factors such as environmental constraints and behavioral habits to form an integrated behavioral model (Figure 6.3).

2.5. *The transtheoretical model and stage of change*

The transtheoretical model and stage of change (TTM) was put forward by Prochaska and Diclemente, two American scholars, in the early 1980s, and has achieved satisfactory results in many practices. TTM is rooted in psychology and describes people's behavioral changes with a dynamic

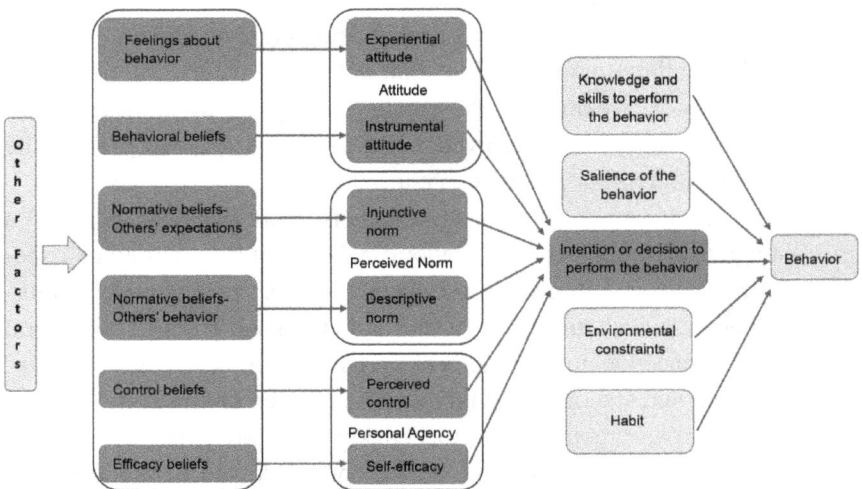

Figure 6.3   Integrated behavior model.

process. The main basis of this theory is that human behavior change is a process rather than an event, and each person who changes behavior has different needs and motivations. By providing different intervention assistance to satisfy people's needs, this can educate them to change toward next stage and eventually adopt healthy behaviors. This is different from several other theories, because other theories explore the causes of behavioral change from behavioral triggers.

TTM believes that human behavior change is a complex, gradual and continuous process, generally divided into five stages, and there is a sixth stage for addictive behavior (Table 6.2).

(1) Pre-contemplation
At this stage, people have no intention to change their behaviors. The reason for the lack of intention may be ignorance of the consequences of

Table 6.2 Behavioral and psychological characteristics of behavioral change phase model.

Behavioral change stages	Behavior plan	Behavioral and psychological characteristics
Pre-contemplation	No intention to change behavior in the next 6 months, or even insist on not changing	Not aware of the existence of problem behavior; or tried to change, but lost confidence because of failure
Contemplation	Intended to change the problem behavior in the next 6 months	Aware of the existence of problem behavior, and the benefits and costs of behavioral change, in a state of contradiction
Preparation	Will change behavior in the near future	Specific plans have been made for the actions to be taken
Action	Behavior changes have taken place in the past 6 months	Behavior changes need to meet criteria that are sufficient to reduce the risk of disease
Maintenance	Adhere to healthy behavior for more than 6 months to achieve the intended purpose	More confident in avoiding temptation and preventing the return of old behavior
Termination	Termination of addictive behavior	No longer tempted, highly confident in the maintenance of behavioral changes

behavior, or numbness in perception, or frustration due to repeated attempts to change but ultimately failure, and so on. Therefore, this unmotivated group often finds some reasons to resist behavioral intervention. For example, they think that behavioral intervention is a waste of time, or that they do not have the ability to make behavioral changes, and so on.

(2) Contemplation
People at this stage have plans to change their behavior, but they have not shown signs of action. They are aware of the potential benefits of behavioral change, but they also know the cost involved, so they are in a conflicting mindset between the benefits and the cost. This stage may not be very long and is often referred to as the chronic intention or behavioral procrastination stage. Stages 1 and 2 are collectively referred to as the pre-preparation phase.

(3) Preparation
People at this stage tend to take action in the near future (usually within a month). They are committed to making changes and taking action, such as developing action plans, finding information, and seeking advice.

(4) Action
People at this stage have made behavioral changes in the past (usually within the past six months). It should be noted that not all actions during this period are behavioral changes. People's behavioral changes must reach the level of risk reduction recognized by professionals. For example, in the behavioral change of safe sex behavior, occasional use of condoms does not count as a qualified behavioral change.

(5) Maintenance
People at this stage have maintained their behavioral state for more than six months and have achieved the desired goal of behavioral change. This maintenance can generally last from 6 months to 5 years if it can withstand temptation and increase self-efficacy. But if they don't withstand the temptation, or if they don't have enough confidence and perseverance, they may return to their original state of behavior. This phenomenon is called relapse.

(6) Termination
For addictive behavior, people at this stage are no longer tempted and have high confidence in maintaining behavioral change. Although they

have negative emotional experiences, such as depression, anxiety, nervousness, they are less likely to relapse. Generally 20% of people can reach this stage.

People at different stages, as well as the transition from the previous stage to the next, will undergo different psychological changes. From pre-contemplation to contemplation, the main experience includes the re-recognition of the original unhealthy behavior, the generation of anxiety and fear, the new understanding of the healthy behavior advocated around and the realization of changing unhealthy behaviors. From contemplation to preparation, people mainly experience self-reevaluation and realize that they should abandon unhealthy behaviors. From preparation to action, people have to experience self-liberation, from cognition to behavior change, and eventually make a commitment to change. Once people start to act, they need many supporting conditions to promote action, such as establishing social support networks, changes in social atmosphere, eliminating events that promote recurrence of unhealthy behavior, and incentive mechanism, and so on.

Behavioral intervention should first determine the stage of the target population, understand the different needs of people at different stages of behavior, and take targeted interventions to help them move on to the next stage in order to achieve the desired results. At the first and second stages, emphasis should be placed on encouraging people to think about and recognize the hazards of dangerous behaviors, to weigh the advantages and disadvantages of changing behaviors, and to generate the intention and motivation for changing behaviors. At the third stage, they should be urged to make decisions and start to change health-threatening behaviors as soon as possible. At the fourth and fifth stages, they should change the environment to eliminate or reduce temptation, and support behavior through self-reinforcing and learning to trust. If the intervention is not ideal or unsuccessful, the behavior of the subject will stay on a certain stage or even go backwards.

People have a series of changes in psychological activities in the process of behavior change, so health educators can take different psychological interventions to improve the effectiveness of behavioral intervention. These methods include:

(1) Awareness-raising: this involves awareness of causes, outcomes, and behavioral therapy for specific problems.

(2) Emotional relaxation: role-playing, witness of successful cases can effectively alleviate the negative emotions, which appear in the early stages of behavior change.

(3) Self-reassessment: this process combines cognitive assessments and emotional assessments of self-images, whether related to unhealthy behavior or not, such as the image of idle individuals and dynamic sports lovers.

(4) Reassessment of the environment: to assess how the existence and absence of individual behavior would influence the emotion and cognition about social environment.

(5) Self-liberation: it refers to the belief that an individual can change and make an effort, and strive for that belief again.

(6) Providing social opportunities and choices: especially for those who are relatively poor and vulnerable. For example, setting up smoke-free areas, providing convenient access to contraceptives.

(7) Mutual social relations: mutual care, trust, frankness and acceptance, and support for healthy behavior.

(8) Reverse constraints: choosing healthy behaviors to replace harmful ones, such as using relaxation, and desensitization therapy to quit smoking.

2.6. *Group dynamics theory*

The group dynamics theory was first put forward by Kurt Lewin, an American German, in 1939. The theory holds that a person's behavior (B) is the result of the interaction between internal needs (P) and external forces (E), which can be expressed by functional $B = f(P, E)$. The so-called group dynamics theory is to discuss the effects and influences of various forces in the group on individuals. Lewin believes that after people form a group, individuals will interact and adapt to each other constantly, thus forming group pressure, group norms, group cohesion, and so on, which not only influences and regulates the behavior of individuals in the group, but also ultimately changes the behavior of the group.

The group dynamics theory mainly includes five aspects:

(1)   Group cohesion

Group cohesion refers to the attraction of a group to its members and the mutual attraction among group members. It is a combination of forces that act on all members and promote their participation in group activities. Group dynamics generally describe cohesive groups as members working together for a common goal, and each member is willing to share responsibility for the group and consistently oppose external attacks. Giving individuals a common task, creating a friendly atmosphere of cooperation among members, members with the same background and attitude, frequent contacts and exchanges, and common encounters or misfortunes are all factors that form group cohesion. In a group with large cohesiveness, individuals have strong collective consciousness, good interpersonal relationships, and strong group behavior.

(2)   Group pressure and group norms

Group norms refer to the code of conduct formed by the group and the members of the group to abide by. They may be explicit provisions such as codes and norms, or they may be unwritten and conventional conceptual frameworks. Group norms can constrain the behavior of individuals in a group and also contribute to group cohesion. And group pressure refers to an atmosphere formed in the group, which makes the individuals have to act in accordance with the group norms keep in line with the vast majority of the group. There are three explanations for the consistency of the group. Group coherence can be explained in three ways. One is that the group as a whole largely determines the thoughts and actions of individual members. The other is that each individual tends to act like other members of the group. The third is that the coherence of individual actions with group members is influenced by the pressure of seeking common ground. There are two main types of pressure for seeking common ground in a group: one is the inherent pressure when a person finds that his or her opinions and behaviors are different from others. The other is the external pressure exerted by members who try to influence the behavior of others. Since these pressures are directly lead to the consistent behavior of group members, they are often attributed to group norms.

(3)   Individual motivation and group goals

Any group will have a goal, which is a reason for existence and action. The goals selected by the group largely determine the behavior of the group, how it works, the dependence of the members on the group, the attitude and confidence of the members, and so on. Research has shown that group goals are closely related to the individual motivations of members, and members who wholeheartedly accept group goals will show the strongest demand motivation demand and work hard to make the group achieve its goals.

(4)   Leadership and group performance

The literacy of leaders and their leadership style play a very important role in the life of all groups. In group dynamics, leadership is generally studied as a function of the group, which involves the exertion of group performance and the level of group productivity. In addition, the study of leadership styles will help solve the problem of how to mobilize the inner vitality of group members.

(5)   Group structure

When a group gains a stability in the arrangement of its members, it also has a certain structure. Group structure variables include formal leadership, roles, norms, status, group size, and group composition. The group structure shapes the behavior of group members, making it possible to explain and predict most of the individual behaviors within the group as well as the performance of the group itself. The group includes normal members, abnormal members, leading members, and isolators. Among them, normal members accept and abide by overwhelming majority of the group's norms, and abnormal members accept some of the norms and reject one or more of them. But they are still members of the group. The leading members make the greatest contribution to maintaining the unity of the group, while the isolated ones are basically not part of the group and usually yearn for another group.

Group dynamics theory can be fully used in health behavioral intervention based on schools, enterprises, institutions and communities. For example, when the intervention of salt intake of elderly hypertensive patients is carried out in a community, if the intervention is decentralized to an individual, which means every elderly person with hypertension, the enthusiasm of the elderly is not high. Firstly, they lack the awareness of excessive salt intake. Secondly, if each elderly person controls the salt intake alone and lacks supervision and encouragement from others, it is often difficult to adhere to and easy to give up halfway. At this time, if all the elderly in the community who are over 65 years old and have high hypertension, that is, individuals with similar age and health problems, are grouped together and organized into an elderly hypertension group to carry out salt intake intervention of the group, the effect is much better than that of individual intervention. In this group, the target salt intake is less than 6 grams per day. Since the goal set by the group is the behavioral orientation of all members, the majority of the members of this elderly hypertension group will actively support and participate in the group's target behavior and this becomes their own conscious behavior. Group members often have close relationships with each other. The elderly in this group are very close because of their similar age and illness experience. In this group, each member has a sense of belonging and a sense of collective honor. In such a group environment, individuals who take the lead in changing behaviors, that is, those who are the first to successfully control daily salt intake below 6 grams, may become the backbone of the group. They can play a positive role in demonstrating to the other elderly people with hypertension in the sick group and can lead others to join salt control actions. At the same time, group members will be constrained by group norms. That is to say, the elderly in the disease group will be constrained by group norms (the daily salt intake is less than 6 grams). They should be consistent with other elderly people. Consistently, if they fail to achieve their goals, group pressure may be formed. This combination of support and pressure can effectively promote the formation of healthy behaviors and change the risk behaviors of individuals in the group. It also means that the pressure and support in the disease group can promote all the elderly hypertensives in the disease group to adopt salt-limited healthy behavior and change unhealthy behavior of salt intake. Introducing the mechanism of competition and evaluation among groups as well as using group cohesion can encourage group members to form and consolidate healthy behaviors, to encourage members with good behavioral interventions, to supervise individuals with gaps, and ultimately to achieve collective health promotion. For example, in the disease group, we can select salt control stars in the disease group, reward the elderly who have reached the salt intake control standard, supervise the elderly who have not yet reached the salt intake control standard, and encourage them to learn from salt control stars. Finally, the goal of collectively reducing salt intake can be achieved among the members of the elderly hypertension group, which leads to the realization of salt intake control.

Chapter 7

Health Education, Health Promotion, and Health Management Process

Health promotion and intervention is a complex systematic project involving the quality of life and life protection of the target population. It covers many aspects of individual, group and social cultural factors that affect health, as well as policy and organizational structure. Therefore, health promotion requires scientific, thorough and systematic planning and evaluation. Health promotion and intervention practices follow a certain basic framework. In short, there are three questions to answer when making a plan[1]:

(1) What is the objective of the plan? It is about clarifying needs and priorities to make goals and objectives clearer.
(2) What will the plan do? This is the process of refining the steps. Specifically the following are included:

Choose the best way to achieve the goal;
Identify the resources to be used;
Set a clear action plan, including who will lead? What to do? How to work together? When to do?

(3) How do you know if a plan is successful? This is the assessment step, and an integral part of the health promotion intervention plan, that needs to be considered before the plan begins.

---

[1] Scriven, A. (2009). *Health promotion — practical guidance* (F. Wei, Trans.). Hangzhou: Zhejiang University Press.

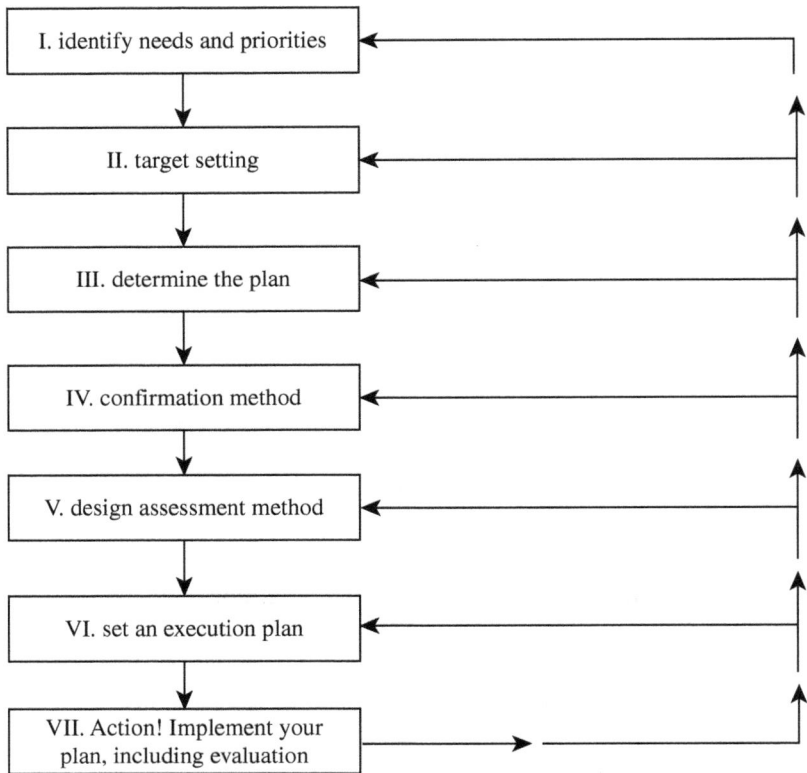

Figure 7.1   Flowchart of health promotion program assessment.

Figure 7.1 outlines the seven steps of the health promotion program assessment process. First, set goals based on identifying needs and priorities; then determine the plan, confirm the method, and design the evaluation method according to the target. Implement the plan (including evaluation) after setting the execution plan. It is worth mentioning that the arrows of the flow chart go around because it is possible to discover something that needs to be rethought when starting the action and adjust the original idea. For example, the original goal was too big and needed to be scaled down; or some resources are not available and need to be adjusted, and so on. The planning process is not always orderly. For example, think about goals (step 2) before thinking about methods (step 4) and if you realize that you can't get the resources you want, you go back to step 2. In this way, a feasible plan can be made and implemented.

The following six principles should also be followed when designing health education and promotion programs:

(1) Principles of purpose: The plan should have a clear general goal and feasible specific goal, so that the plan design has a clear direction, and the plan activities should be carried out closely around the goal to ensure the realization of the plan goal.

(2) Principle of integrity: Health education and health promotion programs are part of the overall health development system. In formulating health education and health promotion plans, not only the health education or health promotion project should be fully understood and considered, but also the consistency of the project with the overall health development plan should be considered.

(3) Principle of forward-looking: When making plans, it is necessary to foresee the future, be advanced to a certain extent, and consider the long-term changes of population needs, resources, environment, and other conditions.

(4) Principle of flexibility: Make room for the plan when making the plan, and adjust the plan according to the actual situation during the implementation to ensure the smooth implementation of the plan.

(5) Principle of reality: In the design of the plan to learn from the experience and lessons of other projects, carry out research, understand the actual situation. Only a plan designed according to the actual situation can truly meet the needs of the target population.

(6) Principle of participation: All groups and institutions involved in the plan should participate in the planning, such as target groups, partners, investors, health educators, and so on.

In the long-term practice, people have gradually formed a systematic framework or model of health promotion intervention. Among them, PRECEDE-PROCEED framework proposed by Lawrence W. Green, a famous American health education expert, in the 1970s, has been widely adopted and become the most widely applied and authoritative guiding framework in the past decades. This framework is also known as the green

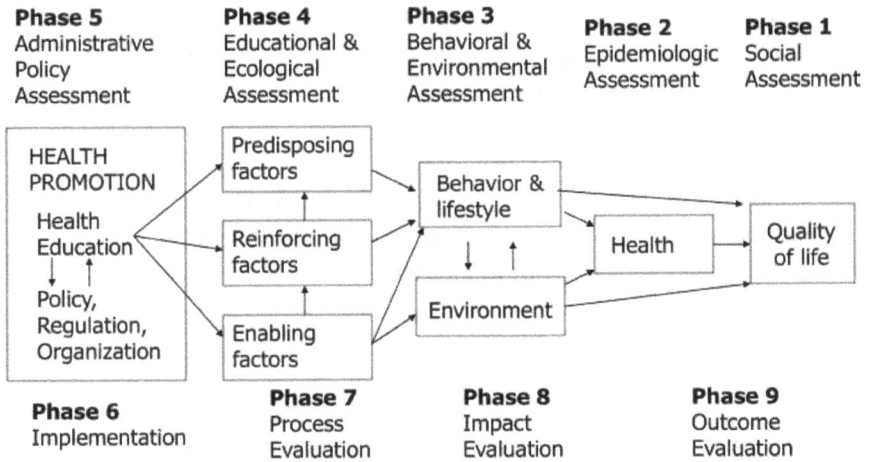

Phase 5	Phase 4	Phase 3	Phase 2	Phase 1
Administrative Policy Assessment	Educational & Ecological Assessment	Behavioral & Environmental Assessment	Epidemiologic Assessment	Social Assessment

HEALTH PROMOTION

Health Education

Policy, Regulation, Organization

Predisposing factors

Reinforcing factors

Enabling factors

Behavior & lifestyle

Environment

Health

Quality of life

Phase 6	Phase 7	Phase 8	Phase 9
Implementation	Process Evaluation	Impact Evaluation	Outcome Evaluation

Figure 7.2　PRECEDE-PROCEED framework.[2]

framework (Figure 7.2). PRECEDE-PROCEED framework offers successive steps of plan design, implementation, and evaluation. PRECEDE is the acronym of predisposing, reinforcing, and enabling constructs in educational/environmental diagnosis and evaluation, it refers to the application of propensity, enablement, and reinforcement factors in education, environmental diagnosis, and assessment. PRECEDE focuses on diagnosis and needs assessment. And PROCEED is the acronym of policy, regulatory, and organizational constructs in educational and environmental development, it refers to the use of policy, regulatory, and organizational tools in education and environmental interventions. PROCEED focuses on the execution and evaluation processes.

Next, we will illustrate the steps of health promotion planning and evaluation with PRECEDE-PROCEED framework.

1. Needs assessment

According to PRECEDE-PROCEED framework, needs assessment includes social assessment, epidemiologic assessment, behavioral &

---

[2] Simons-Morton, B. G., Greene, W. H., & Gottlieb, N. H. (1995). *Introduction to health education and health promotion* (p. 128). Long Grove, IL: Waveland Press.

environmental assessment, educational & ecological assessment, and administrative policy assessment.[3]

1.1. *Social assessment*

Social assessment refers to the diagnosis of the quality of life of the target community or population and the major health problems that affect the quality of life. Social assessment involves understanding the social, economic, cultural environment, health-related policies, and community resources of the target society or population. The quality of life reflects the objective state and subjective feelings of the life of the target population, such as per capita income, housing conditions, environmental quality, health services, and satisfaction with personal quality of life. And the analysis of the social environment including understanding and evaluation of social politics, economy, culture, services, and resources, such as those by social and economic development level, education level, people advocate of faith and belief, customs and habits, the distribution of health resources, utilization of health services, and so on, and service to make the feasible health promotion plan.

Social assessment can be made by a variety of social science research methods, such as in-depth interviews, focus groups, and surveys. It is also possible to obtain useful information about social assessment through secondary analysis of various data provided by health authorities (such as disease surveillance data, maternal and child health records, etc.). The assessment of the quality of life of social groups is usually obtained directly from the population through quantitative methods such as questionnaire survey. The questionnaire can be designed by referring to the existing recognized quality of life scale, and can also be designed according to the actual local conditions or specific research problems. Social assessment must also attach great importance to the qualitative research reflecting the subjective feelings of the masses and social needs. The common methods are: (1) insiders forum: invite community health-related administrative leaderships, health industry experts, community workers, relevant organizations and mass representatives, and other people to

---

[3] Changchun. (2010). *Health education and health promotion*. Beijing: Peking University Medical Press.

provide information about community needs; (2) individual interview: invite people familiar with the community to interview, understand the concerns of the masses; (3) using conventional information: for example, incidence, prevalence rate, morbidity R. rate, admission rate, discharge rate provided by the health administration department, and corresponding data were obtained from previous literatures; (4) on-site inspection: go to the community science for field observation; (5) when the above methods are still insufficient, a special questionnaire can be used for sampling investigation, and a general survey can be carried out if conditions permit, but the evaluation method of rapid sociology is advocated.

1.2. *Epidemiological assessment*

After the major health problems affecting the quality of life were identified by social assessment, the main risk factors of health problems were further identified by epidemiologic methods, and the process of intervention in health problems was determined. Usually "5D" index is used, that is death, diseases, disability, discomfort, and dissatisfaction, to describe the physiological and psychological health status of target population.

In epidemiologic assessment, government and health agency statistics (such as disease statistics, health survey data, etc.) are often used for further analysis to determine the prevalence of diseases or health problems, especially the distribution and occurrence characteristics of diseases or health problems in different populations.

Epidemiologic assessment is used to identify the major health problems that affect the quality of life of the target population, including physical health problems, mental health problems, social health problems, and to identify the health problems that need to be addressed first. Focus on assessing the incidence, distribution, intensity, hazards, and so on of these problems.

Epidemiologic data ultimately need to be able to answer the following questions:

(1)   What are the major diseases or health problems that threaten the population?
(2)   How serious is the disease or health problem?

(3) Who are affected by these diseases or health problems? What are the characteristics? Such as age, gender, education level, and so on.

(4) What are the characteristics of the occurrence of disease or health problems? Such as seasonal, regional distribution, duration, and so on.

(5) What diseases or health problems need to be addressed first? Which disease or health problem is most sensitive to health education and intervention? Probably the best benefit?

1.3. *Behavioral & environmental assessment*

The purpose of behavioral and environmental assessment is to diagnose the risk behavior factors leading to the occurrence and development of diseases and health problems. This is to distinguish between behavioral and non-behavioral factors that cause disease or health problems and to intervene against behavioral factors. Take hypertension patients, for example, smoking and a high-salt diet are behavioral factors, while family genetic predisposition is a non-behavioral factor. In addition to distinguishing behavioral factors from non-behavioral factors, it is also necessary to distinguish important behaviors and unimportant behaviors as well as high-variability behaviors and low-variability behaviors (Table 7.1).

The importance of behavior is shown as follows: (1) The degree of relationship between behavior and health problems. The closer the relationship, the more important the behavior. For example, the relationship between high-salt content and the development of hypertension in hypertensive patients has been confirmed by a large amount of evidence from

Table 7.1 Priority intervention behavior identification.

	Important	Unimportant
High-variability	1. The key act of intervention as a target	3. The act of intervening unless there is a specific purpose and resources are sufficient
Low-variability	2. The act of intervening as a target under certain conditions	4. The act of not considering intervention

evidence-based medicine. High-salt behavior is closely related to hypertension. So high-salt behavior is very important for people with hypertension. (2) The frequency of behavior. The occurrence of high frequency, the importance of the behavior is relatively greater. For example, the high-salt behavior of patients with hypertension, if they eat a high-salt diet almost every day, this behavior is more important. If the patient had only occasional episodes of high-salt behavior and not a high-salt intake, it would be of less importance to the patient.

High-variability behavior usually includes the following characteristics: First of all, it is in the development period or just formed; secondly, it has little to do with traditional culture or a traditional way of life; thirdly, there is evidence of successful change; Finally, social disapproval. High-variable behaviors with several (or some) of these characteristics, if closely related to health problems, should be the focus of targeted interventions. For example, a patient with high blood pressure usually has the habit of smoking, but he does not smoke for a long time, the amount of daily smoking is not large, and smoking is not a traditional culture or lifestyle, smoking is also widely disapproved by the society, and among his friends, there are successful cases of quitting smoking. So, for this patient with high blood pressure, smoking behavior is a high-variable behavior. Characteristics of low-variable behaviors include: behavior has been formed for a long time; deeply rooted in traditional culture or a traditional way of life; there are no instances of successful change in the past. For example, a patient with high blood pressure usually has the habit of smoking, he has been smoking for more than 20 years of history, at least a pack a day, not smoking is uncomfortable, had quit smoking before, but did not succeed. He worked as a salesman, often offering toasts, and his friends were all smokers. No one in the crowd had ever quit. So, for a patient with high blood pressure, his smoking behavior is a low-variable behavior. Of course, under certain conditions, important but low-variability behaviors can also be used as intervention target behaviors. Less important high-variability behaviors can also be intervened if they are adequately resourced and have a specific purpose. But low-variability behaviors that are not important are generally left alone.

1.4. *Educational & ecological assessment*

Health intervention and promotion strategies require behavioral and environmental factors. Factors influencing health-related behaviors, including individuals, small environments, and social environments, which can be inspired by education and organizational structures. For example, health beliefs and health literacy directly determine individual health behaviors, and the formation of health beliefs and the improvement of health literacy cannot be separated from the improvement of social and cultural environment and effective health education. Educational & ecological assessment is the analysis of factors that affect behavior, including tendency, facilitation, and reinforcement. Tendency factor is the motive, desire, or inducing factor of a certain behavior, including knowledge, belief, attitude, values, and so on. Facilitation factors, also known as actualization factors, are the factors that make the motivation or desire of an action come true, including the technology and resources necessary to realize the change of behavior. It happens before the action happens. Reinforcement factors are the factors that stimulate the maintenance and development of behaviors, including social support, peer influence, evaluation of people around, personal feelings after the adoption of behaviors, and so on, which occur after the occurrence of behaviors.

1.5. *Administrative policy assessment*

Administrative policy assessment is the analysis of policies and resources within the organization that may promote or interfere with the development of health education and health promotion projects, including: resources needed and available for the proposed intervention project, organizational impediments or enablers that affect project implementation, available policies or policies that must be changed. The core of management and policy diagnosis is organizational assessment and resource assessment, and understanding of the status of existing policies. This includes the analysis of the establishment of health education institutions and the degree of the government's criminal investigation department's resources investment in the project, and the adjustment with the relevant organizations. This assessment can be carried out by means of expert consultation, qualitative investigation, and data reference.

PRECEDE model divides the diagnosis into five steps, which does not mean that the five steps must be followed completely. Health education personnel can fully adjust the process according to the actual situation. For example, through literature research and expert interviews, educators have completed epidemiologic assessment and behavioral and environmental assessment, followed by social assessment, educational and ecological assessment and administrative policy assessment.

2. Implementation of health education and promotion plan

The sixth stage of PRECEDE-PROCEED framework is the execution stage. The implementation work includes: setting the overall and specific goals of the plan, establishing the implementation schedule, controlling the quality of the implementation, establishing the implementation organization, equipping and training the implementation staff, equipping and purchasing the required equipment and items, and so on.

2.1. *Set the overall and specific goals of the plan*

Based on the above five diagnoses, health promoters were able to set clear goals for health promotion. Among them, the overall goal of the plan is the expected final result after the execution of the plan. For example, in the behavioral intervention of cardiovascular diseases, the overall goal is to reduce the incidence of hypertension and cardiovascular diseases caused by improper diet. This goal is macro and long-term. It's usually broken down into specific objectives. Specific objectives need to follow the principle of SMART, which is specific, measurable, achievable, reliable, and time-bound. Setting specific objectives requires answering the following questions:

Who — For whom (i.e. target population)?
What — Change what to achieve (knowledge, beliefs, behavior, results, etc.)?

When — How long will this change be implemented?
Where — To what extent is this change implemented?
How much — How much change to implement?

Take, for example, "reducing the incidence of hypertension and cardiovascular diseases caused by improper diet". For whom? That is, the target population is the population with unreasonable diet structure in a certain community. What needs to be realized is that they should change their dietary knowledge, build up the belief that they can change the unreasonable dietary structure, put it into action, establish the behavior of healthy diet, and finally hope to reduce hypertension and cardiovascular diseases caused by the unreasonable dietary structure in this community. When can be set in this community within 2 years to achieve this change, the length of time set can be increased or decreased according to the difficulty of specific objectives and the power of investment. Where: to achieve goals within this community. How much change to implement: it could be set to reduce the proportion of people in the community who have an unhealthy diet by 50%, or it could be more specific, such as increasing salt intake by 50% for people who have less than 6 g of salt.

2.2. *Target population segmentation*

Target population refers to those who need intervention in health education and promotion. It is usually divided into the following three groups in the implementation plan:

- Primary target population: people who need direct intervention to promote health. For example, patients and potential patients with Alzheimer's disease (AD) in the community. For people with severe Alzheimer's disease who lack decision-making skills, the primary target group should be their caregivers or guardians.
- Secondary target group: refers to the group that has an important influence on the primary target group, such as relatives, friends, community workers, and so on.

- Tertiary target population: refers to people who have an important impact on the implementation of the project, such as policy makers, community leaders, sponsors, project partners, and so on.

In addition, the target population can be divided into the high-risk population, key population, and the general population according to the severity of the health problems, and health education and intervention can be carried out according to different grades to achieve the effect of promoting health. High-risk group usually refers to the group with the high-risk factors of some diseases, such as people who are obese, tend to eat greasy foods, are inactive, and have a history of diabetes among their first-degree relatives are at high risk for diabetes, they are the high-risk group when doing health education of diabetes. Focus groups usually refer to children, adolescents, women, elderly groups, and so on.

2.3. *Health promotion strategies*

Medical communicators, who are led by medical staff, should combine their advantages and adopt reasonable educational strategies in health promotion. In the era of highly developed media technologies, the "omni-media" strategy of integrating various media technologies provides a good solution for effective health promotion plan. This includes not only traditional health promotion through printed media (including pamphlets, flyers, etc.), interpersonal communication (e.g., peer education, individual guidance, etc.), and community activities (e.g., community lectures, etc.). It is also possible to consider promoting long-term behavior change for target groups through modern new media technologies, such as social networking (WeChat community).

3. Effectiveness evaluation

Evaluation is a systematic process of collecting, analyzing, and expressing information, which is a comparison between objective reality and expected goals. It runs through the whole process of health education and health promotion project management. Evaluation is to understand the effects of health education and health promotion programs; Overall inspection and control of the project; to ensure the advanced planning and implementation quality to the maximum extent. Health promotion programs like other systematic programs, need to be evaluated to prove their value. But unlike other programs, health promotion programs are based on the health behavior of the target population. The results of the evaluation are used to determine whether the goal is achieved and whether it is used appropriately and effectively.

Depending on the nature of the health promotion program, different criteria can be used to determine the value of the health promotion program. These standards include[4]:

(1) Effectiveness: The degree to which the purpose and objectives of the plan are achieved.
(2) Appropriateness: The degree to which interventions are related to demand.
(3) Acceptability: The degree to which the content or method is accepted.
(4) Efficiency: How much time, money and resources will be spent to improve efficiency.
(5) Equity: The balance between demand and supply.

Several common evaluation methods include:

(1) Cost-effectiveness analysis
Cost-effectiveness analysis measures whether it is the most economical way to achieve results, and whether the allocation of resources is reasonable.

(2) Cost-benefit analysis
Cost-benefit analysis is the analysis of the cost of each benefit. Because evaluating health outcomes is difficult in itself, people compare health promotion projects horizontally, it is compares the cost-benefit ratio of one project with some other projects. In general, prevention is cheaper than cure.

---

[4] Yujinming. (2013). *Health behavior and health education.* Shanghai: Fudan University Press.

(3) Diversity evaluation

The success of health promotion plans has different meanings for different groups and stakeholders. Therefore, an ideal approach is to collect data representing the opinions of different stakeholders and form diversified evaluations.

The following will introduce the implementation of evaluation in detail.

3.1. *Types and contents of evaluation*

3.1.1. *Form evaluation*

(1) Related concepts

Forming evaluation is the process of providing information for the design and development of health education programs. This includes provides basic information for the needs of development of intervention plans and the design and implementation of the plans. Its purpose is to make the health education plan in line with the actual situation of the target population, make the plan more scientific and perfect.

(2) Specific contents include

Understand the basic characteristics of the target population.

Find out what the target population thinks about intervention.

Understand education materials distribution system.

Pre-survey and modify the questionnaire.

To understand the suitability of intervention strategies and health education materials.

Adjust the plan appropriately for early problems.

(3) Methods and indicators

Methods included: review of literature, archives, materials; expert consultation; panel discussion; target population survey; field observation; pilot study, and so on.

Indicators include: the scientific of the plan, the supportability of the policy, the suitability of technology, the acceptance of strategies and activities by the target population, and so on.

3.1.2. *Process evaluation*

(1) Related concepts
Process evaluation starts from the beginning of the health education program and runs through the whole process of program implementation. To effectively ensure and promote the success of the project, to evaluate the project performance, and to modify the project plan.

(2) Implementation methods include
Field observation
Survey and interview of community and target population
Hold a meeting of project workers

(3) Evaluation indicators
Development status: implementation and coverage of intervention activities
Participation status: exposure to intervention activities
Effective index of intervention activities:
Effective index = exposure to the intervention/percentage of expected participation

(4) Quality control
Internal quality control: project internal staff strictly grasp the evaluation standards when conducting process evaluation.
External quality control: quality control of process evaluations by outsiders with project evaluation experience, such as panel reviews. Early implementation is especially important.

3.1.3. *Effect evaluation*

(1) Related concepts
Health education aims to improve people's health conditions and quality of life by changing their health-related behaviors. Effect evaluation is to evaluate the changes in health-related behaviors of the target population caused by health education programs and their influencing factors (tendency factors, contributing factors, and reinforcing factors).

(2) Evaluation includes
Tendency factors

Contributing factors
Reinforcing factors
Health-related behavior

(3) Effect indicators include
The average score of health knowledge
The qualified rate of health knowledge
Awareness rate of health knowledge (accuracy)
Incidence of behavior
Rate of behavior change

3.1.4. *The significance of evaluation*

(1) Ensure the quality of plan design and execution
(2) Scientifically explain the value of the plan
(3) Use plan implementation results to gain support and expand influence
(4) Enrich the theoretical knowledge and improve the practical level
(5) Improve the work of professionals

3.2. *Contents and indicators of effect evaluation*

Due to the difference in the sequence of the above effects after the implementation of health education intervention, the health education effects were divided into short-term effects, medium-term effects, and long-term effects.

3.2.1. *Short-term effect evaluation*

The short-term effect is the first health education effect after the implementation of health education intervention, which is usually manifested as the cognitive change of the target population.

Such as the increase of health care knowledge, the change of health concept, the operation skill of realizing health behavior, and so on.

Common indicators of short-term effectiveness include:

(1) Health knowledge score and average score. Such as children's nutrition knowledge score.
(2) The qualified rate of health knowledge. Such as the qualified rate of hypertension knowledge.

(3) Awareness rate of health knowledge. Such as diabetes knowledge rate.

(4) The formation rate of belief (attitude). Such as the formation rate of consciousness in regular physical examination.

(5) Mastery of behavioral skills, such as smoking cessation skills mastery rate, reasonable motor skills mastery rate.

3.2.2. *Mid-term effect evaluation*

The medium-term effect is the behavior change of the target population and the change of policy and environmental support conditions after the short-term effect is achieved. These changes need to be based on improved knowledge and skills of the target population at all levels.

For this reason, the time produced should lag behind the short-term effect.

Common mid-term effect evaluation indicators include:

(1) Prevalence of behavior. Such as smoking rate, breastfeeding rate.

(2) The change rate of behavior. Such as smoking cessation rate, improvement of compliance with hypertensive drugs.

(3) Changes in policies and environment. Such as AIDS policy and environment, health service conditions, technology and other aspects of change, as well as the changes in the atmosphere of public opinion.

3.2.3. *Long-term effect evaluation*

The long-term effect refers to the improvement of health status and quality of life of the target population after the implementation of health education and health promotion programs.

Indicators for long-term effect evaluation include:

(1) Physiological and biochemical indicators of the target population, such as blood glucose control rate and overweight rate.

(2) The cure rate for diseases, such as tuberculosis.

(3) Incidence, such as Incidence of hypertension, the number of reported cases, and so on.

3.3. *Evaluation design scheme*

The following two commonly used project effectiveness evaluation schemes are introduced.

3.3.1. *Pretest and post test of no control group*

It refers to the measurement of relevant effect indicators of the target population before the implementation of health education and health promotion intervention, and then implement the intervention. After all the intervention activities were completed, the relevant effect indicators of the target population were measured again. The results of two measurements were compared to obtain the changes of various indicators, so as to show the effects of health education and health promotion after the implementation of the project.

The advantages of this scheme are simple operation, time-saving, and labor-saving. However, since the design scheme cannot exclude the influence of non-intervention factors, only when the non-intervention factors remain unchanged before and after the intervention, the effect of health education can be accurately reflected.

This scheme is suitable for evaluating the effect of health education project with a short period and stable environment.

For example, for the education of hypertension knowledge in a certain community, the awareness rate of hypertension knowledge in the community was measured first before the education, and the awareness rate of hypertension knowledge in the community was measured again after the education. That's how you compare pretest and post test of no control group.

3.3.2. *Pretest and post test of the control group*

This also known as quasi-experimental study, is designed with the idea of setting the target population as the intervention group and selecting another comparable population as the control group for the target population.

Before the intervention on the target population, the intervention group and the control group were measured. Then health education and health promotion intervention were only given to the intervention group, while the control group was left in a natural state. At the end of all interventions, the relevant indicators for both groups were measured again. Two-way comparison was made between the two measurements to determine the effect of health education and health promotion.

In this protocol, the intervention group and the control group were not randomly determined, but were selected with matching method when they were similar in major factors.

This kind of research is easier to carry out than experimental research, and has the advantages of experimental research.

The scope of application is wide, especially for intervention research projects.

For example, obese people in one community were selected as the intervention group, and obese people in adjacent communities with similar environmental and living conditions were selected as the control group. The prevalence of hypertension and diabetes was measured in both groups. Obese people in the first community were then given health education and health promotion measures about obesity, while the second community was left in its natural state. The prevalence of hypertension and diabetes in both groups was measured again after months and years of observation. This is the pretest and post test of the control group.

3.4. *Factors affecting the authenticity of effect evaluation*

Factors influencing the evaluation refer to several factors that may affect the authenticity of the evaluation results. These factors may interfere with the intervention effect, but they are not intervention factors, which need to be analyzed in the evaluation or overcome through quasi-experiment.

3.4.1. *Historical factors*

Events other than interventions that occur during the implementation of a project, including within national, regional, or organizational structures. Or events that occur at the intervention site, leading to certain changes in participants that may have an impact on the outcome. Such as patriotic health campaigns, world no tobacco day activities and related news reports, which are also called natural changes or long-term trend changes. Such as periodic changes in disease incidence that can be set up control group and process tracking to eliminate the impact of these factors.

3.4.2. *Proficiency of project personnel and participants*

Increased knowledge and changes in skill among participants and staff during the study period also affected the survey results. For example, as the participants grew older, their social psychology became more mature. The members of the control group were repeatedly investigated some knowledge and content, which led to the improvement of cognition. Due to repeated investigation, the staff are more familiar with the investigation content, more skilled in technology and improve the quality of the investigation. This bias can be minimized through, for example, enhanced technical training of staff.

(1) Measurer factor
A measure's intended or unintentional cues to the target population; the evaluation standard is not uniform; not correctly understanding the meaning of indicators; maturity of the measurer.

(2) Measurement tool factor: measurement tool is not accurate.
(3) Measuring object factor: the maturity of measuring the object.

3.4.3. *Lost to follow-up*

Lost follow-up means that during the experiment, the study subjects may migrate, go out, refuse to continue to participate in observation, or die from other causes unrelated to the disease. Non-random loss of follow-up or excessive loss of follow-up in the intervention group or control group can cause bias. When the target population has a high proportion of lost follow-up (more than 10%) or non-random lost follow-up, that is, only the people with certain characteristics lost follow-up, the evaluation results will be affected.

4. Process of health management

Health management aims to prevent and control the occurrence and development of diseases, reduce medical expenses and improve the quality of life. Health education to individuals and groups could improve self-management consciousness and level. The process continues to improve through health information collection, health testing, health assessment, personalized monitoring management program, health intervention, and other means to manage lifestyle-related health risk factors.

Health management was first proposed in the United States in the late 1950s. The insurance industry in the United States has found that most healthy people spend very little of their medical expenses and a small number of people spend most of their medical expenses. It is necessary to identify those who are likely to spend more and take steps to reduce their medical expenses. Therefore, insurance institutions and medical service institutions work together to apply health management technology to identify high-risk groups in the early stage, and through health management to improve the health condition of the policyholder, reduce the risk of illness of the policyholder, reduce medical expenses and insurance company compensation costs, so as to control the risk for the insurance company.

China introduced the concept of health management at the end of the 20th century. Since 2000, under the influence of the United States, Japan, and other countries, the health management industry with health examination as the main form began to rise. In 2001, China's first health management company was registered and established. In order to promote the standard, orderly, and sustainable development of health management industry, China has successively introduced a series of measures in the aspects of health management team construction, health management discipline construction, and health management industry development.

At present, the main way of health management and health service in China is health examination. There are three main types of institutions providing health management services. First, physical examination centers established by medical institutions or health management centers established by their physical examination centers can provide health examination, post-examination analysis, disease intervention, and detection, health consultation, and other services. Second, the community health service center provides health education, early screening, and disease management services for residents with chronic diseases such as hypertension, diabetes, and tumor. Third, the physical examination center or health management center run by the society provides health examination, post-examination consultation, health education lectures, health care, and recuperation and other services.

Currently, health management services in China are mainly applied in the following fields:

(1) Health insurance. In 2004, China insurance regulatory commission issued five professional health insurance company preparation approval, among them, the people's health insurance company of China was the first to be allowed to open in 2005, a number of professional health insurance companies followed. Health insurance companies have formed a "health security + health management" business philosophy and consensus. Establish a set of increasingly perfect health management services with a certain degree of market acceptance, including health examination, health records management, health risk assessment, health intervention and disease management, medical cost management, and other services.

(2) Health management of employees or individuals. More and more domestic enterprises and public institutions begin to realize the importance of employee health for the core competitiveness and development of enterprises. Many enterprises and enterprises provide a regular physical examination for employees, and some enterprises carry out a health assessment, health intervention, and promotion after physical examination for employees, and implement health management projects in the workplace. In addition to enterprises and institutions, many individuals also began to attach importance to their health, will regularly make appointments for their physical examination. Therefore, many physical examination centers came into being, and large hospitals have set up physical examination centers to serve these enterprises and individuals.

(3) Community health services. The functional orientation and service connotation of community health service in China have reflected the concept of health management, such as: health record management of community residents, health examination of key population, early screening of chronic diseases and intervention management of high-risk subjects, follow-up management of patients with clearly diagnosed chronic diseases, group and individual health education, and health

management services in combination with family doctor contract. For example, the elderly in the community for fecal occult blood screening; long-term follow-up and management of blood pressure or blood glucose in patients with diagnosed hypertension and diabetes; the knowledge education and popularization of chronic and common diseases should be carried out regularly for the community population. These are the health management aspects of community health.

4.1. *Connotation and characteristics of health management services*

The connotation and characteristics of health management service include ten characteristics in two aspects.

4.1.1. *That is: comfort, system, continuity, privacy, and feasibility of the service*

(1) Comfort: the environment of health management service is comfortable, warm, and tension eliminated.
(2) System: health management is not a single organ or a single disease, but an endless cycle of services.
(3) Continuity: According to the health status of different life periods to carry out analysis, assessment, monitoring. Make health warning tips, health intervention, health guidance, and health tracking. Only by constantly updating and adjusting health intervention programs can we achieve the purpose of maintaining and improving health.
(4) Privacy: Health management service involves an individual's physiology, psychology, society, family, morality, and other aspects. It is important to protect their privacy so that they can truly expose their health problems in order to effectively develop intervention plans and mobilize and enhance their active participation in health management.
(5) Feasibility: Health management services should always follow the wishes of those served and their feasibility should be fully considered. Only in this way can the service providers accept and actively participate in the implementation so that the continuation of the service will not be hindered.

4.1.2. *That is: scientific, information, diversification, humanization, personalized service*

(1) Scientific

The transition from health to disease is a complete evolutionary process that is assessed on the basis of a wealth of health and disease data, biological clinical indicators, and evidence-based medicine and disease-related diagnostic guidelines.

Scientific evaluation of individual health risk factors and hierarchical management can optimize the effect of health management and have substantial management significance.

(2) Information

In the process of health management, advanced information technology can make management services more convenient. Health information and health management services are available anytime and anywhere. Through the use of disease prevention and control information management to achieve health information resources sharing, it is of great significance to improve the efficiency of health management services and medical treatment.

(3) Diversification

Health management service is the multi-dimensional and multi-layer intervention management of human health. Each individual has different health needs due to his or her different physique. In order to meet the basic needs and special needs of the people served, a diversified service program can be established so that everyone can participate in and enjoy health management services.

(4) Humanization

Health management services emphasize "people first", focusing on people rather than disease. This is a complete break with previous medical conventions. It embodies the humanistic emotional color of the service, so that the service more friends or partners of intimate service.

(5) Personalized

The impact of different health risk factors on health and the risk of disease and intervention measures vary from individual to individual. At the same time, the dimension and frequency of health intervention are also different, so as to improve health better and more effectively.

4.2. *Health management strategy*

The basic strategy of health management is to maintain health by assessing and controlling health risks.

Health management strategies include lifestyle management, needs management, disease management, disaster injury management, disability management, and comprehensive population health management.

Factors that affect human health include:

Environmental factors: environmental factors include natural environment, psychological environment, and social environment. Natural environment includes primary environment (original natural environment) and secondary environment (artificial modified natural environment). Psychological environment includes personality, stress and life stress factors, emotions, and so on. Social environment includes economic income, living conditions, nutrition, culture, and so on.

Lifestyle and behavior factors: lifestyle is formed in the process of socialization and under the mutual influence of people. A good lifestyle contributes to health, while a bad lifestyle or even deviating from behaviors such as smoking or drinking can do harm to health.

Biogenetic factors: biogenetic factors are the basis for understanding life activities and diseases.

Medical and health service factors: medical and health service is a kind of social measure to control diseases. The layout of medical and health service, the allocation of resources, the policy of a healthy work, the level of technology, and the quality of service all have a direct impact on people's health quality.

4.2.1. *Lifestyle management*

Lifestyle management is the basic component of health management strategy and can be integrated into other health management strategies. An individual's behavior or lifestyle may pose certain health risks that affect the individual's health care needs. Lifestyle management helps individuals change unhealthy behaviors, adopt healthy behaviors, reduce health risk factors, and reduce the risk of disease and death. Lifestyle management requires the mobilization of individuals' sense of responsibility for their own health, and the promotion of behavior change through the application of four intervention techniques, either alone or in combination:

(1) Education: transfer knowledge, establish attitude, and change behavior. Educational interventions are an essential component of most lifestyle management strategies. Traditional health education methods focus on changing knowledge and attitudes rather than individual behavior. The goal of lifestyle management is to improve health. Individualized education programs are a very effective way to educate patients on self-management of chronic diseases. The disease management program focuses on the combination of clinical and chronic behavioral management, while the lifestyle management program focuses on educating patients on how to manage their own situation.

(2) Incentives: incentives are also called behavior modification. Incentives can be successfully corrected by applying the knowledge gained from theoretical learning to change the relationship between the environment and behavior. Behavior modification can be divided into six categories: positive reinforcement, negative reinforcement, feedback promotion, punishment, feedback consumption, and elimination.

(3) Training: Through a series of participatory training and experience, individuals are trained to master behavior correction techniques. Consists of six sections, lectures: teaching examples of technology being properly used in the classroom; Demonstration: describe the technical behavior in detail; Practice: participants practice new techniques by hand; Feedback: the trainer provides the trainees with the feedback information of behavior moderation and validity; Reinforcement: provide rewarding feedback, such as verbal praise or material rewards; Homework: encourage individuals to practice new techniques after class through homework.

(4) Marketing: use social marketing and health communication technologies to promote healthy behaviors, create a healthy environment, and promote individuals to change unhealthy behaviors. Social marketing is to make people accept social ideas and change their behaviors through celebrity effect. Health communication programs include market analysis, market segmentation, marketing strategy, raw materials and product distribution, training, monitoring, evaluation, management, schedules, and budgets. Health communication activities are increasingly using mass media. PSAs and TV storylines are used to inform the public about health risks and healthy behaviors.

Lifestyle management has two characteristics:

(1) Focus on the individual
It emphasizes that individuals should be responsible for their own health, arouse their initiative, and help them make the best choice of healthy behaviors.
Assess the health risks associated with an individual's lifestyle or behavior and the impact of health risks on the individual's health care needs.

(2) Focus on prevention
Lifestyle management helps individuals change behavior, reduce health risks, promote health, and prevent disease and injury. Prevention includes primary, secondary, and tertiary prevention, with the emphasis on primary prevention.

4.2.2. *Demand management*

Demand management is one of the common strategies of health management, including self-care service and crowd diversion service. Its essence is to help management objects maintain their health and seek appropriate health services, control health costs, and promote the rational use of health services. The goal of demand management is to reduce the use of expensive, clinically unnecessary health care services while improving the health of the population. Demand management can be used to properly use medical care services to meet their health needs by telephone, Internet and other means to guide management objects, such as seeking alternative therapies for surgery, helping patients reduce specific risk factors, adopting a healthy lifestyle, encouraging self-care, and so on.

Four factors obviously affect people's medical consumption demand.

(1) Prevalence rate: reflects the level of disease in the population.

(2) Perceived need

An individual's view of the importance of the disease and whether they need to seek medical care. This is the most important factor affecting the utilization of health services.

Including: personal knowledge of the risks of disease and the benefits of health services, personally perceived efficacy of recommended therapies, personal ability to assess the problem, personal perceived severity of the problem, personal ability to deal with the problem independently, and personal confidence in dealing with the problem well.

(3) Patient preference

The important role of patients in medical service decision-making is emphasized. The doctor's job is to help patients understand the benefits and risks of such treatment.

(4) Motivation other than health factors

People's ability to take sick leave, disability benefits, co-payments in insurance, and sickness benefits can all influence their decision to seek medical care.

Methods and techniques for demand forecasting include:
- Questionnaire-based health assessment;
- Assessment based on health care costs.

Common needs include: 24-hour call triage service, referral service, internet-based health information database, health class, service appointment, and so on.

4.2.3. *Disease management*

Disease management is another major strategy for health management. The American institute for disease management defines disease management as "a system that coordinates healthcare interventions and communication with patients, emphasizing the importance of patient self-care. Disease management supports doctor-patient relationships and health care programs, emphasizes evidence-based medicine and individual empowerment strategies to prevent disease progression, and evaluates clinical, human, and economic outcomes based on sustained improvements in individual or group health". Disease management emphasizes the importance of patient self-care which is essentially patient self-management. Patients must monitor their progress and improve their behavior in various areas, such as medication adherence, diet, and symptom monitoring. Patients must communicate their illness status to health care professionals on a daily basis. Patients with chronic diseases are less likely to repeat visits after being taught how to manage their disease.

Disease management includes "crowd identification, evidence-based medicine guidance, physician and service provider coordination, patient self-management education, predictive management of process outcomes, and regular reporting and feedback".

The target population of disease management is individuals with a specific disease. It does not focus on individual cases and their single visit to the doctor, but focuses on the continuous health status and quality of life of individuals or groups, and emphasizes the importance of integrated coordination of health services and interventions.

4.2.4. *Management of catastrophic injuries*

Management of catastrophic injuries is a special type of disease management that, as its name implies, focuses on "catastrophic" diseases or injuries. "Catastrophic" can mean a serious health hazard, or it can mean a huge medical and health cost, such as tumors, renal failure, or severe trauma. Catastrophic injuries are very serious injuries that require particularly complex management, often requiring multiple services and relocation of treatment sites. Because the availability of services is greatly affected by family, economy, and insurance, the incidence rate is low, and long-term complex medical and health services are required, the management of catastrophic injuries is more complicated and difficult than the management of ordinary diseases. It requires a high degree of specialization to help coordinate medical activities and manage multi-dimensional treatment programs to reduce medical costs and improve health outcomes. To maximize clinical, financial, and psychological outcomes for patients with catastrophic injuries.

While common chronic diseases are predictable in terms of intensity and effect, catastrophic injuries are relatively rare, and their occurrence and outcome are difficult to predict. Catastrophic injuries management can reduce costs and improve outcomes by coordinating medical activities and managing multi-dimensional treatment programs. Through a comprehensive use of patient and family education, patient self-care choices, and multidisciplinary team management, patients with complex medical needs can maximize clinical, financial, and psychological outcomes. Catastrophic injuries management relies on specialized disease management services to address relatively rare medical problems and high costs.

Good management characteristics of catastrophic injuries include: timely referral; comprehensive consideration of various factors, the development of an appropriate medical service plan; having a team with multiple medical specialties and comprehensive business capabilities to effectively respond to the various medical service needs that may arise; maximize patient self-management; patients and their families were satisfied.

4.2.5. *Management of disabilities*

The objective of disability management is to reduce the frequency and cost of disability accidents in the workplace and, from the perspective of the employer, to deal with disability separately according to the degree of disability to minimize the decline in labor and living capacity caused by disability. For employers, the real cost of disability includes lost productivity. The loss of productivity is calculated in terms of all the costs incurred by the entire replacement workforce. These workers must be used to replace those who are absent due to short-term disability.

Reasons for the different length of disability include medical and non-medical factors. Medical factors include: severity of illness or injury; individual choice of treatment; rehabilitation process; the period of discovery and treatment of disease or injury (early, middle, and late);

the difficulty of receiving effective treatment; drug or surgical treatment; age affects how long it takes to heal and recover, as well as the likelihood of returning to work (older people take longer); the presence of complications depends on the nature of the disease or injury; drug effects, especially side effects (e.g. sedation). Non-medical factors include: psychosocial problems; occupational factors; work pressure; the relationship between workers, colleagues, and supervisors; dissatisfaction with work tasks; psychological factors include depression and anxiety; the information channel of transitional work is not smooth, and so on.

The specific objectives of disability management include the following eight aspects:

(1) Prevent deterioration of disability;
(2) Focus on functional recovery, not just pain relief;
(3) Set expectations for actual recovery and rework;
(4) A detailed description of the constraints and possibilities for future action;
(5) Assess the influence of medical and social psychological factors;
(6) Communicate effectively with patients and employers;
(7) Consider reinstatement when necessary;
(8) Circular management should be implemented.

4.2.6. *Health management of comprehensive population*

The health management of comprehensive population provides a more comprehensive health and welfare management for individuals in the population by coordinating the above five health management strategies. Health management of the comprehensive population should be considered in health management practice.

From the macro health management strategy, the country should focus on health monitoring and disease control from the beginning of disease treatment to the whole process of life. Pay attention to prevention, treat future diseases. National overall health resource management needs an authoritative, unified, coordinated and organized management organization. For every 10% increase in life expectancy, GDP increases by 1.1%.

4.3. *The process of health management*

The service process of health management generally includes the following eight steps:

4.3.1. *Sign customer service agreements*

On the basis of an in-depth understanding of customer health needs, according to their own service ability to meet customer service requirements to the greatest extent possible. To sign a service contract with customers in a practical and realistic way, perform duties according to the contract, and be honest and promise to deliver the service.

4.3.2. *Collecting health information*

It is a reliable basis for health risk analysis and evaluation to collect health-related information through the health information questionnaire survey and physical examination data. The content of the questionnaire survey is determined based on the health needs of the population and based on the principles of early detection and early intervention, and can be adjusted according to the individual's gender, age, job characteristics, or the relevant characteristics of the group.

4.3.3. *Establish a complete health record*

Establishing health records is necessary for health management. Health records are used to record a client's vital signs and any health-related behaviors and events they have engaged in. Health-related information was collected through questionnaire survey and physical examination on individuals or groups, and personal health records were established on this basis.

4.3.4. *Conduct health risk assessments*

Based on the health-related information (questionnaire and physical examination information including personal basic information, family history, past history, lifestyle, mental stress) collected, the health risk factors of individuals or groups, and the risk of disease or death in the future were assessed. Provide a series of assessment reports, including personal physical examination report, personal overall health assessment report, mental stress assessment report, and so on These are quantitative indicators for the development of health intervention plans and programs.

The health risk assessment process is as follows:

(1) Health screening

Health managers collect information about the health and lifestyle of individuals or groups. And find health problems. And differences in health risk across gender, age, risk factors, predisposition to disease, and high risk of death. Design health checks for different age groups. A periodic health assessment can accumulate continuous health information for individuals to help them make effective health decisions and maintain their health.

(2) Analysis and assessment of the future risk of illness and death

The core of health risk assessment is to predict the case fatality rate or prevalence rate of the population with certain characteristics in a certain period of time in the future according to the principles and technologies of evidence-based medicine, epidemiology, and statistics.

Health information and physical examination report of the managed population were analyzed and judged by health managers and experts based on scientific data indicators through evaluation software and consultation discussion.

(3) Quantitative evaluation

This is an important feature of health risk assessment, that is, assessment results are quantifiable and comparable. Common HRA assessment results include risk of disease, health age, health score, and so on.

The basic idea is to convert the calculation result of health risk into a numerical score through certain methods.

(4) Risk management

Identify risks, evaluate risks, select risk management methods, implement, and feedback.

(5) Write a risk assessment report

Risk assessment reports are written and given by health management professionals.

4.3.5. *Develop health intervention plans and programs*

Based on the assessment of the existing health risks, the control objectives and risk reduction intervention plans and programs are developed.

After health risk assessment, health counseling and other health management services are provided to individuals. Customers can make an appointment with the health management service center for consultation, or communicate over the phone. The service mainly includes explaining personal health information, health assessment results and their impact on health, making personal health management plans, providing health guidance, and making follow-up plans.

4.3.6. *Implementing health interventions*

Based on health management intervention plans and programs, a step-by-step approach in a variety of forms helps individuals take action to correct poor lifestyles and habits, control health risk factors, and achieve the goals of the individual health management plan.

4.3.7. *Health dynamic tracking*

Follow up the personal health management plan through SMS, phone, Internet, email, door-to-door, and so on, and conduct regular re-evaluation to provide the latest improvement results to individuals, so that health can be effectively managed and maintained. It is more important to keep abreast of the client's physical changes and health status to continuously adjust and revise health intervention plans and programs.

4.3.8. *Effect evaluation of health management*

In the process of management, periodic effect evaluation and annual effect evaluation are given to customers' health status, such as the evaluation of individual intervention and comprehensive intervention effect, the improvement evaluation of lifestyle before and after the intervention, and the improvement evaluation of behavioral factors.

In addition to the above routine health management services, special health management services can be provided for individuals or groups according to the actual situation. For individuals with chronic diseases, services can be provided for specific diseases or risk factors, such as hypertension management, diabetes management, cardiovascular disease-related risk factors management, mental stress relief, smoking cessation, exercise, nutrition and dietary counseling, and so on. For individuals without chronic diseases, services such as personal health education, life-style improvement counseling, and education and maintenance of high-risk groups can be provided.

4.4. *Implementation steps of health management*

The implementation steps of health management usually include the following aspects:

4.4.1. *To accept the service*

Including visits, telephone inquiries, online questions and other services before joining the health management, as well as relevant services that have become the official customers of the health management agency, and the acceptance of the services or questions that should be received.

4.4.2. *Receive counseling*

The content of health management service, the benefits brought to the other side and the scope of service are described in detail. Staff should be warm and generous, clear service objectives, tone and voice close and gentle, but not servile, vague, secretive, casual commitment.

4.4.3. *Collect basic information about personal health*

Collecting the basic information of personal health means obtaining relevant information and requirements through various ways. Information gathering is the first and critical step in making information available. The quality of information collection is directly related to the quality of the whole information management.

4.4.4. *Establish health records*

Health records management includes: home page of health records, personal health information form, abstract of medical history, previous health examination report (individual, group), latest health examination report (individual, group), records of health testing and monitoring indicators, records of health management dynamic tracking, dietary management diary table, sports management diary table, records of health consultation and feedback, record of expert consultation and intervention service, health management services, record of appointment service execution, and so on.

4.4.5. *Design of health examination items*

Design of health examination items: according to different ages, different people, different nature of work to personalized design. To carry out a personalized, targeted and timely design. Done by a health management specialist or health manager.

4.4.6. *Arrange and make an appointment for physical examination*

Make arrangements and appointments in advance. The health manager is responsible for filling in the "appointment service notice", coordinating with the physical examination center to arrange services, and informing the target population of the date of physical examination arrangement.

4.4.7. *Identify and achieve the objectives of physical examination*

Physical examination: follow the medical examination service procedure. After the completion of physical examination, the participants should be informed of when to retrieve the physical examination results, the time required for expert analysis and evaluation, appointment arrangement and interview for tentative time, and so on And timely fill in the "Records of health management dynamic tracking" and "A list of prescribed treatments". After the physical examination report is retrieved, the physical examination results shall be timely notified to the group undergoing the physical examination, and an appointment shall be made for the interview time. After the service, health management experts fill in the "record of expert consultation and intervention service", "Records of health management dynamic tracking" and "A list of prescribed treatments".

4.4.8. *Summary and analysis of physical examination report*

Summary and analysis of the physical examination report shall be completed by professionals from the final examination report department and health management department of the physical examination department. The summary and analysis of the physical examination report should be considered from two aspects: one is the possibility and diagnosis of the presence or absence of disease in the clinical body state; the second is whether there are health risk factors and predicting the future development trend of body health.

4.4.9. *Comprehensive analysis and evaluation of health risk factors*

Based on the basic information of personal health and comprehensive indicators of the physical examination report, scientific, objective and comprehensive analysis, and evaluation of integrity are made.

4.4.10. *Development of a "guidance manual on health risk assessment"*

Analyze the risk factors of body health. Develop health management intervention plans and health guidance implementation plans through analysis and evaluation. Propose specific management service measures to improve individual health. Provide information about what to change, motivate and desire, provide ways to do it, get healthy behavior changes, and so on. Develop a guidance manual for health risk assessment (guidance program for health management interventions).

4.4.11. *Develop a phased implementation plan and program for health management*

(1) Initial management objectives: The primary criteria for management improvement, that is the priority problem to be solved, should be the health problem that can be improved in the short term and has a significant effect. Specific implementation plans and solutions should be proposed for the main problem.

(2) Medium-term management objectives: to evaluate the effectiveness of the improvement of key issues, to comprehensively adjust minor issues, and to propose specific implementation plans and solutions.

(3) Quarterly and annual management objectives and effect evaluation: According to the assessment of the implementation and implementation of the above management objectives, the physical condition will be re-examined comprehensively and the results before and after will be compared and evaluated. The improvement should be maintained, and the new health problems should be timely supplemented. Revise and adjust the management intervention plan to achieve maximum health change and health promotion.

4.4.12. *Health management services were officially launched*

The health management process of the target population is as follows: acceptance service, reception consultation, health file management, health physical examination, health assessment, health guidance, first consultation after health assessment, initiation of health management procedures, and systematic health management services.

4.5. *Comprehensive health management and service system*

Comprehensive health management service system usually consists of eight systems, three mechanisms, eight parts, and six services.

4.5.1. *The eight systems*

Comprehensive health management integrated system

(1) Health electronic records management system. This is the power of health management.
(2) Health examination management system. This is the source of health management.
(3) Health management assessment system. This is the core of health management.
(4) Health management intervention system. This is the embodiment of health management.
(5) Health management payment system. This is the health management budget.
(6) Health management coordination system. This is health management support.
(7) Customer service management system. This is health management feedback.
(8) Health management tracking system. This is the effect of health management.

4.5.2. *The three mechanism*

4.5.2.1. Maintenance mechanism — first-level management

(1) Health maintenance.
(2) Health care.
(3) Health promotion.

4.5.2.2. Conditioning mechanism — secondary management

(1) Reverse subclinical.
(2) Control abnormal indicators.

(3) Psychological stress reduction.
(4) Health preservation in Chinese medicine.

4.5.2.3. Comprehensive rehabilitation mechanism — three-level management

(1) Common diseases.
(2) Chronic diseases.
(3) Comprehensive treatment.
(4) Rehabilitation.

4.5.3. *The eight parts*

(1) Analysis and evaluation of current health status.
(2) Health risk assessment and intervention.
(3) Chronic disease risk prediction.
(4) Health guidance implementation plan.
(5) Exercise guidance program.
(6) Dietary guidelines.
(7) Health education and psychological counseling.
(8) Comprehensive medical care.

4.5.4. *The six service*

(1) Health examination service.
(2) Dynamic management service of health records.
(3) Routine medical care service.
(4) Health intervention management expert service.
(5) Medical green channel service.
(6) Health education and publicity services.

In the west, health management programs have become a very important part of the health care system and have been shown to be effective in reducing individual risk and health care costs. Health management experience in the United States has shown that participants in health management services are 50% more likely to take prescribed medications regularly and

60% more likely to report more effective drugs and treatments with effective proactive prevention and intervention, thereby reducing the overall risk of participants in health management services by 50%. However, in China, health management is still a new concept. The service object of health management is relatively narrow, mainly concentrated in the population with high economic income. The public awareness is not enough, and some ideas of health management have not been accepted by the public. However, through the efforts of professionals, it is believed that health management will be gradually accepted by people. Health management is not only a concept, but also a method and a set of perfect service procedures. Its purpose is to enable patients and healthy people to better recover, maintain and promote health, and save expenditure, effectively reducing medical expenses. The authorities predict that "the 21st century is the century of health management"! Health management not only can reduce the cost of medical expenses and the length of hospital stay, but also can reduce the health risk factors of the managed. Health management is a chronic process, but the return is huge.

Chapter 8

Cases of Medical Communication to Specific Populations: A Case Study of Osteoporosis

Osteoporosis (OP) is the main risk factor of causing fragility fractures. This kind of disease has become a troublesome problem of public health, making an impact on the society, health, and economy. The main symptoms of osteoporosis include pain, functional limitations, and changes of patients' life quality. Due to the higher life expectancy and population aging trend, there is a very high incidence rate of osteoporosis in China. In the prevention of osteoporosis, the main purpose is to prevent fragility fractures. In that case, we should pay more attention to the following points: (1) promote bone formation in adolescence, making people gain enough peak BMD; (2) lay more emphasis on the bone loss problem in adulthood, especially after menopause; (3) keep bone health all the time; and (4) prevent falls.

There are enough factors to prove that multi-factor tests (which includes risk evaluation, healthy living habits, smoking cessation, moderate alcohol consumption, outdoor physical training, sun exposure, and balanced diet) are effective for the high-risk group of osteoporosis. There are some tips for osteoporosis prevention: (1) increase the intakes of calcium, phosphorus, magnesium, cesium, and fluoride; (2) take enough vitamin D (even from fortified food); (3) eat more foods with Omega(ω)-fatty acid; decrease the intake of salt and reheated-meals; and (4) take protein properly. In the absence of lactose intolerance, consumption of milk and dairy products, especially yogurt and dairy products with added vitamins, would also be helpful.

1. Influencing factors of osteoporosis

Primary osteoporosis is a kind of systemic bone disease, which is shown as decline of bone mass and destruction of bone tissue microstructure, which will lead to an increase in bone fragility and cause a significant increase in the risk of fracture. Primary osteoporosis is one of the common diseases in the middle aged and the elderly, especially females. As China's population is aging, the number of patients suffering from osteoporosis is increasing. Since the disease is still lacking effective treatment, the social problems caused by it are increasingly prominent. Therefore, in that case, in-depth studies of the etiology of primary osteoporosis are very important to formulate prevention methods. Current research suggests that endocrine hormones, lack of physical exercise, diet and lifestyle, vitamins, mineral elements, and genetic factors are closely related to the occurrence of osteoporosis. Orathai *et al.* believe that osteoporosis is also related to body mass index (BMI), age, fracture history, family history of osteoporosis, and whether eating foods containing beans, dried beans, and grain. The negative correlation between BMI and osteoporosis should be carefully considered. The higher BMI people have, the lower the risk of osteoporosis. Contrarily, it will cause a higher hazard of overweight related diseases. Wang Yuhuan *et al.* believe that gender, characteristic of past job, income, and medical security are the main factors affecting the health behavior of elderly people with high-risk osteoporotic fractures, and the educational level is the main factor affecting the health behavior of elderly people with low-risk osteoporotic fractures. Sleep disorder is one of the most common symptoms of the elderly, which is caused by the sleep anatomy part that produces lesions or physiological functional disorder. It will cause symptoms such as abnormal sleep and excessive sleep. Sleep disorder is one of the most common symptoms in the elderly. Chronic ache caused by osteoporosis is the direct cause to the sleep disorder of the elderly. Wang Ye *et al.* believe that the improvement of mental and physical state of the elderly will improve the quality of those patients with osteoporosis. Encouraging the elderly to insist on doing proper sports program every day, to quit smoking and drinking, and to develop good sleep habit can improve the sleep quality of the elderly. The prevention of osteoporosis is to control the cause. Hormone regulation, nutritional status, living habits, physical factors, immune function, and genetic genes all have effect on the occurrence of osteoporosis. Among these factors, the genetic factors are uncontrollable, and hormone regulation (estrogen replacement therapy) is used during menopause. Nutritional status, living habits, and physical factors can be achieved through intervention.

2. Living habit

2.1. *Aspects of drug dependence*

Both good living habits and reasonable medical treatment are important for the prevention and treatment of osteoporosis. However, patients have poor compliance in clinical, especially in the long-term treatment. Those patients who do not finish the continuous chronic disease management may suffer some serious complications such as spinal compression fractures and hip fractures. Scholars from home and abroad are all starting to explore chronic disease management measures of osteoporosis to improve patients' compliance of medical treatment and reasonable lifestyle. Winzenberg *et al.* propose courses for osteoporosis prevention and self-management. Tamaki *et al.* compile an evidence-based guideline for the prevention and treatment of osteoporosis and fractures based on the community health center. Liu Hairong *et al.* establish osteoporosis club for the health education. All the projects mentioned before achieved excellent results. With the development of information technology, Luo Zhanpeng *et al.* raised the model of continuous health management of osteoporosis which based on the digital platform. All these methods can cultivate patients' good living habits and long-term compliance with medication.

2.2. *Aspects of diet and living habits*

2.2.1. *Physical exercise*

Lack of physical exercise can be regarded as a direct cause to primary osteoporosis. Appropriate physical exercise can not only avoid the occurrence of osteoporosis effectively but also improve the level of bone metabolism for OP patients. People who insist on physical exercises always have a low incidence of osteoporosis. It may because that physical exercise significantly accelerates the blood circulation of the whole body bone directly, while the contraction and relaxation of the muscle stimulate the attached bone, thereby increasing the bone density and the bone mass. Decrease in exercises may result in bones lack of proper load, which would be harmful to the improvement of bone strength. What's more, physical exercises can increase the diameter and peak bone mass of the lower limbs. However, the sustained increase in bone mass still requires long-term physical exercise. What needs to be emphasized is that OP patients should follow the principle of gradual progress in their exercise and remember that safety is the most important thing. The blind pursuit of strenuous exercise may lead to some serious consequences, such as fractures.

2.2.2. Dietary

The intake of fats and proteins in the diet can not only regulate the differentiation of osteoblasts but also affect the formation of osteoclasts. High-fat diet can promote osteoclast differentiation and increase the number and biological activity of osteoclasts. Animal experiments show that lipid oxidation products are found in the bone marrow of animals in the hyperlipidemia model group. The lipids are also deposited in the VRS of Haversian canal which indicating that hyperlipidemia has the potential to promote bone absorption. Further research found that activity of osteoclast is synchronously correlated with blood lipid levels. Therefore, people with excessive fat content in the diet are more likely to have osteoporosis. On the other hand, the proteins which make up the bone matrix material can increase the storage and absorption of calcium, which is beneficial to delay and prevent osteoporosis. However, some studies also suggest that excessive intake of protein may hinder the absorption of calcium in the body.

2.2.3. Unhealthy behavior

Referring to those unhealthy behaviors, there are many studies investigating the relationship between smoking, drinking, caffeine, and osteoporosis. The average bone mineral density of people with tobacco and alcohol addiction is significantly lower than those who at the same age but without such addiction. It also shows that the longer the history of tobacco and alcohol addiction is, the more obvious the decrease in the value of bone mineral density, which shows a negative correlation. And for those people who have both two unhealthy living habits, the decrease of bone mineral density is greater than a single smoker or alcoholic. Caffeine intake also increases the risk of osteoporosis. The relation can be showed in two large-scale research works in the United States for the female. Those research works show that caffeine intake can accelerate the excretion of urinary calcium, and more intake may cause lower level of free estradiol in the body, which further exacerbates bone loss. However, some scholars believe that caffeine intake has nothing to do with bone loss in healthy women.

Orathai *et al.* believe that the occurrence of osteoporosis in the elderly is related to smoking and drinking green tea. Smoking is a risk factor for osteoporosis to the elderly. Contrarily, drinking green tea is a protective factor for osteoporosis to the elderly.

NAG believes that excessive consumption of sweets and caffeinated drinks can have a negative impact on bone mineral density, even if the bones have had demineralization. Food and beverage intake is an important factor that cannot be ignored in the treatment of osteoporosis.

Huang Heping believes that calcium is the raw material for bone anabolism. It is also the material basis for the bone growth and the formation of peak bone mass. Adequate calcium intake can prevent the osteoporosis. On the other hand, both drinking and smoking are the risk factors for causing osteoporosis. Excessive both drinking can lead to osteoporosis, which increases the risk of fracture. Nicotine in cigarettes can stimulate the activity of osteoclasts to some extent, so that the concentration of blood calcium and urinary calcium increases, which will cause the bone density to decrease. The length of sunshine time can promote the formation of active vitamin D, which can increase the absorption of calcium and achieve the purpose to increase the bone mass.

Therefore, the living habits of the elderly can be intervened through the health education of osteoporosis. Those effective interventions can be used to slow the progression of osteoporosis and improve the quality of life of the elderly.

3. Aspects of behavioral intervention

Behavior determines health, and more attention should be paid to the male population and low-income groups who would have high risk of experiencing osteoporosis. By using a multi-channel health education approach, different support and help could be provided to the elderly who suffer from different risks with different needs, to minimize fractures, and finally to help save health costs and improve their quality of life. Luo Shuangying believes that proper nursing intervention for patients with osteoporosis can improve the clinical symptoms of patients and improve their quality of life, and also can cooperate effectively with drug treatment. Besides, Guo Lingmei believes that behavioral interventions help patients build healthy lifestyles. Osteoporosis is mainly caused by a lack of exercise in modern civilization, thus developing regular and quantitative exercise plans as well as effective implementation would be quite useful. The mechanical stimulation of exercise can promote the proliferation and differentiation of bone bud cells, and also promote their formation, and regular exercise is also beneficial to maintain bone mass. Outdoor sports can increase the biosynthesis of vitamin D in the body and reduce its loss. Exercise can also promote blood circulation, promote the nutrients supplement for bone tissue which is conducive to calcium storage and bone growth and improves OP symptoms. By enhancing the patient's physical strength through exercise, it can also improve their normal social skills which could in turn further improve life qualities. Meanwhile, Huang Xiufeng and others also believe that good eating habits, adequate calcium and vitamin D, balanced diet intake, and abstaining from tobacco and drink can reduce the occurrence of osteoporosis. Habit intervention could further strengthen the patient's compliance with healthy diet, drug treatment, and by these efforts we could improve patients' symptoms of osteoporosis and their quality of life.

3.1. *The way of comprehensive intervention*

Comprehensive intervention methods include: (1) health education, such as conducting group health education lectures; (2) issuing health education manuals; (3) family visit guidance; and (4) telephone supervision. Comprehensive intervention and simple dissemination of publicity materials both can increase the awareness of osteoporosis among the elderly, but the effect of the previous is just better than the traditional sole dissemination data group. The main reasons are as follows. (1) Researchers pay attention to the use of communication skills during the comprehensive interventions, and adopt various forms of health education methods, such as group teaching, group discussion, and dissemination of brochures. The form of the lectures mainly adopts electronic slides, which are illustrated clearly and are easy to understand. When designing the manual, considering the characteristics of the elderly and the level of culture, the content is designed to be easily understood and well meet the psychological characteristics of the elderly over 60 years old, thus improving the effect of knowledge dissemination related to OP. (2) 80% of the elderly in the intervention group are in marriage. The researchers also pay attention to the education of family members while spreading the knowledge to the subjects, and encourage the family to learn relevant content, so that the whole family are aware of the importance of preventing OP, so they are more prone to taking a healthy and beneficial lifestyle. (3) All the subjects included in the study have been evaluated by FRAx tools which show that they have high risk of experiencing OP fracture in the next decade. The researchers have provided individualized suggestions in the face-to-face family visits according to each subject's risk factors. (4) Through telephone supervision, the memory of the elderly's knowledge about osteoporosis can be strengthened.

Education level, monthly income, daily physical activities, and anxiety are all important factors influencing the self-management health behavior of the OP elderly. The government should focus on the elderly who are with low education level, incapable of handling their daily lives, with low income and high anxiety, and try to take appropriate measures to improve the self-management health behavior of the elderly and promote healthy aging. The intervention of the diversified health education model can play an important role in improving the self-management health behavior among the elderly.

3.2. *Diversified health education model*

The methods of health education should be diverse. In the process of implementing diversified health education interventions for the observation group, we mainly adopt one-on-one health education, organizing health education among elderly people, distributing health knowledge mission manuals, doing family visits and so on.

3.2.1. *Knowledge education*

This mainly includes organizing lectures on osteoporotic fractures. Based on the degree of their acceptance, we should choose a more understandable way to introduce OP-related knowledge, as well as the relationship between osteoporosis and fracture occurrence, including the causes, risk factors, treatments, how to establish a healthy lifestyle, and the prevention of osteoporosis.

3.2.2. *Diet guidance*

More attention should be paid to calcium and other nutrient intake. Calcium is the main component of bone formation, and calcium deficiency will increase the risk of osteoporosis in the elderly, therefore we need to advocate the elderly to have a high-calcium diet, to eat enough calcium-rich foods such as fish, shrimp, shrimp skin, beans, seaweed, bone soup, coarse grains, sesame seeds, melon seeds, green leafy vegetables and nuts, etc., in their daily lives. Daily requirement for calcium for the elderly should be 1000–1200 md. At the same time, it is helpful to receive enough sunshine and get appropriate vitamin D supplementation to help calcium absorption. However, do not blindly intake one or a few trace elements for a long time; watch for the balance among various elements and pay attention to the diversity of recipes, so as to prevent osteoporosis occurrence.

3.2.3. *Exercise guidance*

Exercise could prevent the occurrence of osteoporosis. Increasing the number of daily activities can increase bone mass and maintain its level. Exercise can exert direct mechanical effects on the bone, making the bones strong to avoid fractures. It can also improve the gait and balance ability of the elderly, reducing the fall-causing risk of fracture. Active exercise and weight-bearing exercises such as swimming, walking, jogging, climbing stairs, and dancing could help reduce bone loss and maintain bone mass in old age. Persistence in 45 min per time, 3–4 times per day of weight-bearing exercise can increase bone density and prevent falls by improving the sensitivity and coordination of the body. Moderate and regular exercise is one of the effective measures to prevent osteoporosis. Swimming has the most significant effect on the increase of bone mass among all kinds of sports. The effect is related to the amount of exercise, indicating that the amount of bone mass increases significantly when the amount of exercise is increasing.

3.2.4. *Safety guidance*

For the elderly with osteoporosis, we should strengthen their safety protection guide, improve their coordination of movement. For example, when using the toilet, getting up from the bed, taking a bath, etc., the elderly should stand still before making another move; remembering to hold on the handrails when they get up or down off the stairs, or take the bus. They should also avoid to get to the crowd place, which could prevent collisions. In daily life, the elderly need to wear anti-slip shoes to avoid obstacles, wear comfortable and non-slip shoes to prevent slipping and falling. We also need to prepare crutches for the elderly who have unstable walking and weak limb strength. Family members must accompany them when they go out, while the elderly themselves also need try to maintain a good posture that could avoid weight bearing, use waist circumference if necessary, which is conducive to the prevention of vertebral fractures.

3.2.5. *Psychological guidance*

We should give timely guidance and solve psychological problems according to the different psychological reactions and analysis reasons for the elderly. The disease must be given enough attention due to the psychological burden to the elderly. Although osteoporosis itself does not change greatly, the complications of osteoporosis are more serious. Guiding the patients to treat the disease correctly, to maintain a good mental state and a peaceful mood, to be open-minded and cheerful, all of which could have a big help for disease treatment.

3.2.6. *Medication guidance*

Drugs can prevent osteoporosis occurrence for the elderly. When people get old, meeting their middle age, especially for women after menopause, bone loss would accelerate. During this period, bone mineral density examination should be performed once a year. For people with rapid bone mass reduction, prevention and treatment measures should be taken as soon as possible. Medicine treatment is mainly aiming at abnormalities in metabolism in patients with osteoporosis. Postmenopausal or senile osteoporosis patients have estrogen reduction, loss of bone calcium, and lack of certain vitamins, so estrogen, calcium, and vitamin preparations can be taken to supply the body's deficiency, but the medicine treatment must be performed under the doctor's guidance. Effective treatment measures would be taken to increase bone mass and reduce the incidence of senile osteoporotic fractures.

3.2.7. *Family visit guidance*

One-on-one household guidance to the observation group would be performed. Individualized intervention plans (including calcium intake, diet, exercise) are advised for the specific elderly. We also supervise the progress of the plan.

The dissemination of publicity materials and diversified health education interventions both can improve the OP-related knowledge and health behaviors in the elderly, but the latter one has better effects. The dissemination can be used as an adjunct to comprehensive interventions, not just the only means. The vision and memory of the elderly are also gradually declining, which makes reading more difficult for them, so documents education cannot achieve good results. Only through diversified health education interventions, we can positively change the lifestyle, life attitude, personality, and mood of the elderly, improve the understanding of reasonable diet, increase physical exercise, and change their bad life behavior. By all these efforts, we can significantly reduce the occurrence of accidents such as fractures in the elderly and ensure the safety of the elderly, improve the quality of life of the elderly, then relieve the worries of their families.

Tian *et al.* believe that the risk of osteoporosis occurrence is closely related to the age, postmenopausal age, menstrual suspension, body mass index (BMI), and education level of postmenopausal women. As for older men, osteoporosis is associated with age, BMI, current smoking, alcohol consumption, physical activity, and exposure to sunlight. After adjusting for age, height, weight, and menopausal time, high osteocalcin and c-terminal cross-linked collagen levels were associated with low bone density. However, deficiency of 25(OH)D, serum Ca, and P was not associated with the risk of low bone density.

In short, osteoporosis is a complex disease associated with multiple factors. Its occurrence and development are related to the environment, diet, exercise, age, endocrine system, and various trace elements. Among the drugs commonly used for the elderly such as statins, proton pump inhibitors, heparin, hormones, calcium carbonate + vitamin D3 tablets, results from partial correlation analysis show that only statin lipid-lowering drugs, calcium carbonate + vitamin D3 tablets are related to bone density. Liu *et al.* believe that in addition to gender, weight and bone density, other factors like alcohol consumption, drinking tea or milk, taking statin lipid-lowering drugs or calcium carbonate + vitamin D3 tablets, exercise, etc., also have an independent preventive effect on osteoporosis. Therefore, age, gender, calcium use, smoking, tea and coffee consumption, and weekly exercise frequency are the main factors that affect osteoporosis occurrence among the elderly people. Older age, female, calcium deficiency, smoking, lack of tea or coffee consumption, and lack of exercise are risk factors for elderly osteoporosis. Prevention of osteoporosis should begin from child-hood and continue in adulthood. Although the genetic determinants of muscle and bone may provide other treatment options in the future, experts should now focus on the effects of lifestyle changes, including healthy eating habits and regular exercise. Vitamin supplementation, specifically vitamin D, should be considered according to the needs of the patient. It should be noted that estrogen status is also important. In addition, patients should be instructed to quit smoking and avoid moderate drinking.

4. Summary and discussion

Osteoporosis is a very common disease, especially for the elderly. It can cause great harm to the human body, such as fragility fractures. We often heard that an elderly person accidentally fractured and then passed away quickly. Therefore, osteoporosis must be treated with caution and intervention, especially for the elderly.

To prevent a disease, first, we must understand the risk factors of this disease. This chapter analyzes the risk-causing factors of osteoporosis, including age, body mass index, eating habits, family history, and then explains these factors of osteoporosis from the aspect of living habits, and finally from the behavioral approach, exploring ways to reduce the occurrence of osteoporosis, and coming up with a model of diversified health education.

The model of diversified health education can also be used in medical communication. For people with osteoporosis-related risk factors or those already suffering from osteoporosis, giving them a wide range of medical science education and guidance, and effectively carrying out tertiary prevention of diseases could reduce osteoporosis and slow down its development, which are of considerable benefits.

Part IV

Medical Communication for the General Public

Chapter 9

Medical Communication for the General Public

In addition to the one-to-one medical communication in the clinic (Part II) and the medical communication for specific target population (Part III), a wider range of medical communication occurs between medical staff and the general public. This part begins with the discussion on the demand for the medical science popularization of the general public, and then focuses on this medical communication model through the analysis of the characteristics of the general public.

1. Demand for and current situation of medical science popularization of the general public

As of the end of 2017, China's population reached 1.39008 billion. From the perspective of age structure, the total population aged 0–15 (including that less than 16 years old) is 247.19 million, accounting for 17.8% of the total population; the total population aged 16–59 (including that less than 60 years old) is 901.99 million, accounting for 64.9% of the total population; and the total population aged over 60 years old is 240.9 million, accounting for 17.3% of the total population. Young and middle-aged people dominate the composition of population. Furthermore, according to the *China Statistical Report on Internet Development*, as of June 2018, the number of Internet users in China was 802 million, with 29.68 million new Internet users in the first half of the year, and an increase of 3.8% compared with the end of 2017. The Internet popularity rate reached 57.7%, including 788 million mobile Internet users, accounting for 98.3% of the Internet users. Chinese Internet users are mainly teenagers, young adults, and middle-aged groups. As of June 2018, the 10–39-year-old group accounted for 70.8% of the total Internet users. Among them, Internet users aged 20–29 are the largest proportion, accounting for 27.9%; the proportion of 10–19 and 30–39 years old is 18.2% and 24.7%, respectively, basically consistent with that at the end of 2017. The proportion of middle-aged Internet users aged 30–49 increased from 36.7% at the end of 2017 to 39.9%, and the penetration of the Internet increased among middle-aged people. The population of China is mainly composed of young and middle-aged people. Furthermore, the proportion of Internet users is extremely high in the young and middle-aged population. Correspondingly, their demand for science popularization will be realized through the network.

According to the *Report on the Search Behavior of Chinese Internet Users' Demand for Science Popularization* in 2015, the demand for science popularization of Chinese Internet users has increased by 178% over the past four years, of which the wireless science popularization search index accounted for 67.16% of the total science popularization search index. Health and medical care are the top popular science topics among Chinese Internet users. The top ten hot search words under health and medical topics are cough, cold, vitamin, AIDS, diabetes, pain, diarrhea, health care, infection, and hepatitis B.[1] Furthermore, in the *Report on the Search Behavior of Chinese Internet Users' Demand for Science Popularization* in 2017, top popular science topics search contents were still health and medical care, accounting for 63.16%, which was significantly different from other search contents. Besides, the growth rate of health and medical science topics search index was 43.18%; that also ranked first. The top three hot search words are gastritis, earlobe, and nephritis.

In view of the above data, health is closely related to everyone, and the public is thus generally interested in health and medical information. The general public's demand for medical science popularization is quite

---

[1] Qi, Z., Hu, J., Wu, D., & Wang, L. (2016). *Clarification of the science popularization demand side — data analysis of internet users' science popularization behaviors.* Beijing: Science Press.

huge, and a considerable amount of the population's medical science popularization knowledge is obtained through the network. Of course, a large number of elderly people are not good at using smart phones and networks due to their lack of ability to use high-tech products, and they are likely to acquire medical science knowledge through more traditional means, such as books, newspapers, television, and science lectures.

However, in view of the current situation of medical science popularization, there is still a long way to meet the needs of the people. According to the statistics of the Ministry of Science and Technology in 2012, there are 14,103 full-time science popularization creators, accounting for only 0.72% of the total number of science popularization personnel in China. Human resources for science popularization are organizers and advocators of science popularization activities, disseminators of science and technology, and an indispensable part of science popularization activities. The lack of human resources hinders the development of medical science popularization. Although there are a large number of medical staff in our country, the number of full-time or part-time personnel directly involved in medical science popularization is limited, which restricts the publicity effect of medical science popularization. Moreover, there are few creators of medical science popularization, which is quite disadvantageous for the spread and popularization of medical science popularization. Furthermore, in terms of the publication of popular science books, the publication quantity of popular science books was 7,521 in 2012, 2.26 percentage point lower than that in 2011, accounting for 0.83% of all kinds of books. The proportion of popular science books is quite rare in all books, and medical popular science books are even rarer accordingly.[2] With the enhancement of people's health awareness, many publishing houses are willing to publish medical popular science books. However, there are still some problems in medical popular science books:

(1) Compilation according to the model of medical monograph books. The compilation of medical popular science books follows the

---

[2] Department of Policies, Regulations and Restructuring of the Ministry of Science and Technology of the People's Republic of China. (2013). *Statistics of science popularization in China*. Beijing: Scientific and Technical Documentation Press.

editing model of medical science, which narrates according to etiology, pathology, symptoms, prevention, and treatment, and it has become a simple repetition of medical theory books. It may be hard to understand for the general public without medical knowledge.

(2) Lack of readability and operability. The language is rigid, the arrangement is not lively, and there are few books full of facts and photographs. The contents that readers want to know are quite vague. Therefore, such books are similar in contents and form, and lack personalized features.

(3) Pseudoscience of "harming people without any consideration" and non-science of "harmlessness and uselessness" in medical popular science books. There are many problems in the market of medical popular science books, such as outdated contents, single writing method, few original works, and low circulation. Consequently, there is also a crisis in readers' trust in medical popular science books. Medical popular science books spread the knowledge of medical science, which not only affects people's cognition, but also affects people's life behavior. Therefore, to ensure the scientificity of the content is the basic criterion for the dissemination of medical popular science.

(4) Problems about authors of medical popular science books also exist. There is a lack of professional medical science creators. Medical staff with professional knowledge have no time, energy, or interest to write such books, while some authors of non-medical background write medical and health books extensively. As a result, the guidance on readers is inevitably biased. It is necessary for the author of science popularization to grasp the scientific nature and spread the scientific spirit, or the consequences will be unimaginable.

In addition to the above general situation of science popularization, medical science popularization also has certain particularity. Medical science popularization activities and propaganda forms are relatively single in the past. Today, with the development of network, digital TV, mobile phone, and emerging media, the publicity channels have been greatly expanded, and the promotion and operation of medical science popularization activities are becoming increasingly more diverse. Weibo,

WeChat, and APPs related to medical science popularization not only innovate in the activity form of medical science popularization but also open up the activity space of medical science popularization. It makes full use of new media, we media, and other communication advantages to improve the effectiveness of medical science popularization. However, medical science popularization is different from other science popularization contents after all. It may not be beneficial but harmful to the health of the audiences if the medical contents disseminated are incorrect or defective. At present, there are increasingly more contents of medical science popularization, but the entry barrier of health science popularization production is low; the good and bad products are intermingled, with increased one-time science popularization, less system tracking, and lack of continuous guidance concerning the science popularization works. In the age of information, there is much accessible medical science popularization information around the public. At present, the problem of medical science popularization is not "presence or absence", but "how to win support among the people" and "how to ensure the accuracy and reliability". Although there are also many medical stars like "Zhang Rongya from Beijing Union Medical College Hospital" and "Shrimp Mummy" on various new media and we media platforms, the number of medical workers is still quite limited compared with the massive medical health information. Subsequently, the medical false information and rumors are overflowing. Taking WeChat Subscription as an example, it has also become a disaster area of medical false information and rumors. Various kinds of doubtful information are widely spread under the banner of health information, which may bring harm to people's health and property. The overflow of general health care information on the we media platform is far from the dissemination of professional health knowledge. In fact, the so-called medical science popularization is the rise of the content marketing method of packaged health information.[3] In this regard, with the rapid development of new media and we media, the forms of medical science popularization are becoming increasingly more

---

[3] Li, D. (2016). Who is spreading health in the micro-screen communication era — communication analysis on the rise of health care information on wechat platform. *Modern Communication (Journal of Communication University of China)*, *04*, 21–26.

diverse, and the areas of communication are becoming wider. However, how to ensure the accuracy and reliability of medical science popularization content is still worth exploring.

For example, if a netizen suffers from diabetes and wishes to get medical knowledge about diabetes, he searches for possible relevant knowledge through the Internet, we media, new media, etc. However, this netizen is not a professional in medicine, and does not have the diabetes-related medical knowledge, which means that he has no ability to identify whether the knowledge he searches is correct or not. His search method is more likely to be based on the amount of readings, and he thinks that it may be correct as long as the amount of readings is high. As for whether the knowledge he searched is correct or not, he is not aware. It is likely that the medical knowledge he searched through readings is not correct, but is pseudoscience or advertising information. Under these circumstances, if the search content is followed, the netizen's diabetes will not only be out of control but also may have complications.

2. Medical communication model for the general public

Science popularization is a process of dissemination of information, knowledge, thoughts, and ideas in essence. The disseminated contents of information, knowledge, and others can be traced back to the scientific community led by scientists. However, for various reasons, science popularization has not become the primary task of scientists, and even scientists do not pay attention to science popularization but have prejudice to science popularization on the contrary. Therefore, in the past work of science popularization, mass media or professional science popularization workers need to build a bridge between scientific groups and the public (Figure 9.1).

Science is the study of various kinds of knowledge through detailed classification (such as mathematics, physics, and chemistry) to form a gradually complete knowledge system. It is about the knowledge of discovery, invention and practice, and the general name of the knowledge system for human beings to explore and understand the law of change of all things in the universe. Science is an orderly knowledge

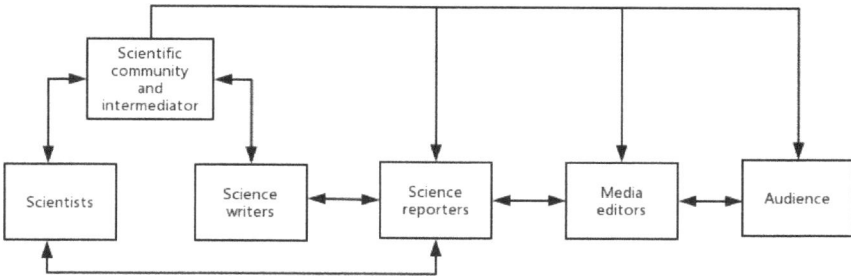

Figure 9.1 Science popularization behavior model.[4]

system based on verifiable interpretation and prediction of the form and organization of objective things. In an old, closely related sense, "science" also refers to the subject itself that can be reasonably explained and reliably applied. The professional practitioners of science are customarily called scientists.

However, due to the limited knowledge of the general public, most of them cannot fully understand science. There is a deep gap between scientists and general public such that the scientific community thinks that the public lacks knowledge and does not strive for progress, while the public also thinks that the scientific community is superior and otherworldly. Misunderstandings lie between the two groups. Therefore, how to spread the extremely profound scientific knowledge to the public through a simple and understandable way is what the popularization of science needs to do. In the past, the scientific community needed to establish a bridge of communication with the public through agencies. Based on the above figure, scientists, science writers, science journalists, and media editors all perform their respective duties and ultimately spread profound scientific knowledge to the public. Here, let's review the concepts mentioned. Scientific community is a collection of scientists with the same scientific concept — the principal component of scientific activities. The task of the scientific community is to establish and develop the best relationship with scientists for acquiring reliable knowledge, which has the norms of universality, public ownership, selflessness, and well-founded skepticism.

---

[4]Nian, Z., & Wang, L. (2015). The concept and classification of science popularization and talents. *Report on the Development of Science Popularization Talents in China*, pp. 34–67.

Scientific writers, as the name implies, are creators of scientific works. Scientists can be scientific writers, but scientific writers are not necessarily scientists. Science journalists are people that are engaged in scientific content and news coverage as well as reporting in the media. Scientists transmit the scientific content to the audience, with or without the scientific community as an intermediator; the transmission process could be via science writers or science journalists as professional science workers, and finally through the editing of media editors. There are many links in the process, and content deviation is easy to appear in the process of transmission.

However, nowadays, with the deepening of the importance attached to science popularization and the increasing control of scientists over the autonomy of public discourse, increasingly more scientists are joining in the science popularization force. Therefore, to a large extent, new scientists could surpass the mass media or professional popular science workers to carry out the medical communication facing the public. As a result, the model of mass-oriented medical communication has changed (Figure 9.2).

From the perspective of the public-oriented model of medical communication, the disseminator is a front-line medical professional with basic medical knowledge, which can guarantee the accuracy and reliability of the medical knowledge to the greatest extent, while the audiences are the general public. The contents of communication between them

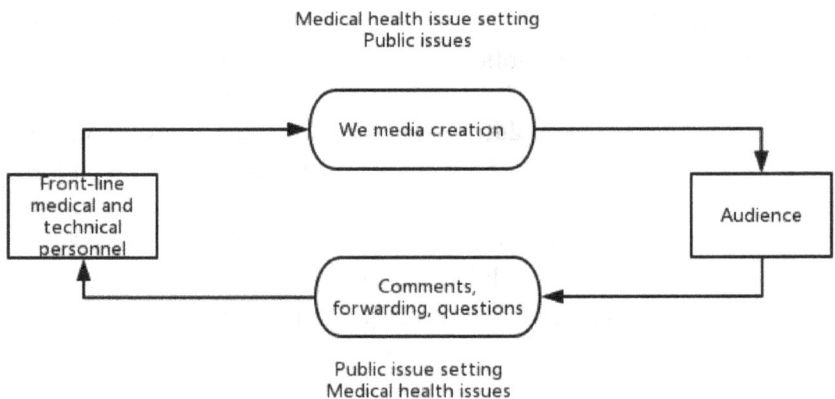

Figure 9.2 Public-oriented medical communication model (self-created).

should be the knowledge of medical health that the public care and need to know. Public topics can be set according to medical health issues, or medical health issues can be set according to public issues reversely. When the topics set are spread to the public through the creation of we media by front-line medical and technical personnel, the public can comment, ask questions, and repost. The comments and questions made by all the general public can be transmitted back to the front-line medical and technical personnel. Furthermore, medical and technical personnel can answer the questions of the public, and understand the public's concerns through the comments and repost of the public, so as to help them better set up topics that the public is really interested in and helpful to them next time.

Let's review some examples. For instance, Valentine's Day is the peak period of marriage and date, and the following month is also the peak period for abortion. Therefore, in view of this phenomenon, some Obstetrics and Gynecology Hospitals and WeChat channels with obstetrics and gynecology content will perform some science popularization and dissemination of contraceptive knowledge, and the setting of this content is in line with the medical health issues concerned by the public at that time. In the process of communication, individuals who read the content can also leave messages and comments in the backstage, and ask questions about contraception. Subsequently, the operators of the WeChat Subscription can answer these questions, and can also make some simple observation and statistics to figure out which part of the public's knowledge of contraception needs to be strengthened or which part requires further improvement, etc., so that they can also focus on the popularization of this aspect in the future. In this way, good interaction and circulation are formed. The disseminators can make their science popularization contents more vivid and practical, and the audiences can grasp some knowledge that can be obtained through science popularization lectures or newspapers and TV without leaving home. At the same time, many people are too shy to consult in contraceptive knowledge, which may lead to improper abortion. Fortunately, the spread of the Internet can ensure that people do not appear in the public, can protect the privacy of individuals, and can obtain the corresponding contraceptive knowledge with protected privacy.

Take children's accidental injuries as another example: during the summer vacation every year, there is a high incidence of children's accidental injuries. Child drowning or traffic injury is frequently reported. According to the characteristics of this period, we media or new media can perform medical science popularization about the prevention of children's accidental injury. Besides, the general public who pay attention to children's accidental injuries can learn relevant knowledge from the science popularization. If they have any question, they can leave a message in the backstage for further consultation, forming a good interaction and communication chain.

3. Three levels of medical communication for the general public

In Chapter 1, we introduced three levels of medical communication: disease, seeing a doctor, and attitude toward disease. In this section, we will detail how to effectively conduct the medical communication for the general public from these three levels.

3.1. *Disease*

Disease can also be called sickness, illness, etc. The occurrence of disease is an extremely complicated process. In many cases, the process from being healthy to being unhealthy is one from quantitative change to qualitative change. When the external pathogenic factors act on the cells, reaching a certain intensity or for a certain period of time, in other words, when there is a certain amount of accumulation of pathogenic factors, damage to the cells may be caused, and the damaged cells may have functional, metabolic, and morphological structural disorders. In the long run, it may lead to a disease.

There are many types of diseases, which can be divided into infectious diseases and non-infectious diseases and can also be classified according to various systems of the human body.

From the prospective of infectious diseases, the infectious diseases are those caused by various pathogens that can be transmitted between humans, between animals, or between humans and animals. In other words, the infectious diseases of someone may be infected by others or animals. In history, there were many major infectious diseases, such as the Black Death in the Middle Ages in Europe. After its outbreak in the Sicilian Islands in 1347, it swept across Europe within three years and killed 25 million people, about half of the people in Europe, within 20 years. The Black Death is actually a plague, which is a fulminating infectious disease that is transmitted from mice to humans and then transmitted from one person to another. However, because people at that time lacked medical knowledge about the plague, and no one told them how to prevent the Black Death, the transmission of the disease was very fast and the mortality rate was quite high.

Then in the era of rapid technological development, what can we do in the field of medical communication in the face of infectious diseases? There are some examples below. It is well known that hepatitis B is an infectious disease caused by hepatitis B virus. There are many hepatitis B patients in China, and about 130 million people are carriers of hepatitis B virus. Many people who do not know the reason may be afraid to talk about hepatitis B. They do not dare to eat, shake hands, or even work together with those who have hepatitis B. Some patients with hepatitis B believe that it is the end of the world and they are in a constant state of anxiety. In fact, hepatitis B is not as terrible as imagined. In this case, we need medical professionals to perform proper medical communication for the general public. The transmission route of hepatitis B is mainly mother-to-child transmission, blood transmission, and transmission by close contact with body fluids. Will we be infected with hepatitis B if we eat, shake hands, and work with hepatitis B patients or hepatitis B virus carriers? The answer is no. However, if a mother is a carrier of hepatitis B virus, then the chances of the baby being born with hepatitis B are very high. Therefore, we, as medical professionals, need to tell people not to worry about working and eating with the hepatitis B virus carriers or to discriminate against them. Hepatitis B virus carriers or hepatitis B patients who are in stable periods can do most of their work with normal people, so we do not have to worry too much. Certainly, if a woman carrying hepatitis B virus is pregnant, it is necessary to go to a regular hospital for hepatitis B virus blocking treatment, so the possibility of carrying hepatitis B virus in a born baby is greatly reduced. In recent years, the number of hepatitis B virus carriers in Chinese newborns has been greatly reduced, which is also very relevant to the publicity and promotion of this knowledge among women of childbearing age.

There are some examples of acute infectious diseases below. For example, influenza is a very common disease and referred to as flu. Many people do not take the flu seriously and think that the flu is the same as a cold. It's hard to image that in history, the Spanish flu between 1918 and 1919 caused about one billion people worldwide to be infected, 25 to 40 million people died (at that time, the world population was about 1.7 billion), and its global average fatality rate is around 2.5% to 5%. Certainly, under today's medical conditions, the flu is far less horrible than it was 100 years ago. Therefore, in the epidemic season of flu, the correct medical communication shall guide everyone to pay attention to the flu, especially for some people with low immunity, such as the elderly, infants, and cancer patients. If you have similar symptoms, you shall go to the relevant hospital in a timely manner, and avoid causing unnecessary panic in the crowd.

In addition to infectious diseases, non-infectious diseases are more common in life, and many people are familiar with diseases such as hypertension, coronary heart disease, and cancer. Chronic non-infectious diseases, referred to as chronic diseases, are a general term for a type of disease that is difficult to identify the cause, has a protracted course, lacks evidence of a contagious biological pathogenesis, and has a complex pathogenesis and has not yet been fully confirmed. Chronic diseases that are mainly controlled in China include cardiovascular and cerebrovascular diseases, cancer, chronic respiratory diseases, and diabetes.

The condition of chronic diseases generally progresses slowly when the body is in good condition, the external factors are controllable, and effective treatments are provided. Otherwise, the disease progresses rapidly when there are factors that contribute to the progression of the disease on the body or when the body is in poor health, and the disease progresses at a rate similar to that of an acute illness, which is called an acute attack of a chronic disease.

Due to the influence of aging of society, unhealthy lifestyles, environmental pollution, and food safety, the prevention and treatment of acute and chronic diseases in China is very serious. In 2016, the number of deaths due to chronic diseases and acute attacks in China accounted for 86.6% of the total number of deaths, resulting in a disease burden accounting for 70% of the total disease burden. According to projections, in 2018, the number of strokes, coronary heart disease, and hypertension in China alone is 13 million, 11 million, and 270 million, respectively. In the next 10 years, the number of patients with chronic diseases and acute attacks in China will continue to grow rapidly, which has become a serious public threat to the health of our people and social development. Therefore, the comprehensive prevention and control of chronic diseases and acute attacks has risen to a national strategy.

Despite the severe prevention and control situation, most chronic diseases and their acute attacks can be intervened and prevented at an early stage. Therefore, in the field of chronic diseases, the application space and significance of medical communication is significant.

There are some examples below.

For example, hypertension is a very common chronic disease in China, and its incidence rate has probably reached about 25% in adults; in other words, one in four adults has hypertension. What can medical communication do for such a large number of hypertensive patients or potential population suffering from high blood pressure? From the concept of three-level prevention of diseases, medical communication can do a lot of work at every level of prevention.

Take primary prevention of hypertension as the first step. Primary prevention refers to the prevention of the pathogenesis. Namely, when there is no disease, intervention of some risk factors is carried out to avoid the occurrence of the disease. From the concept of primary prevention of hypertension, the risk factors for hypertension include high-salt diet, increased fat and calories in food, decreased physical activity, overweight or obesity, drinking, smoking, and mental stress. Therefore, during medical communication, we shall tell people that diet shall be of limited amount of salt, less oil, and low fat. Usually, we need to take proper exercise, quit smoking and drink less, control weight, and maintain psychological balance. Nevertheless, such generalities on science popularization often do not work well. For instance, if we only tell people that they need proper exercise, they will ask what proper exercise is. Everyone has a different understanding of proper exercise. Some people believe that walking a few hundred meters a day is proper exercise, while some believe that proper exercise means running two kilometers a day. Therefore, the correct approach is that we need to tell people what kind of exercise is more suitable, how long it takes to exercise every day, and what kind of amount of exercise is considered proper exercise.

Secondary prevention of hypertension follows. Secondary prevention is preclinical prevention, which means early detection, early diagnosis and early treatment in the early stage of the disease in order to detect and treat the disease at an early stage, avoiding or reducing the complications, sequelae and disability, or shortening the time of disability. For the secondary prevention of hypertension, how often shall a potential hypertensive patient measure his/her blood pressure, and how to determine whether it is hypertension after the blood pressure rises, how to evaluate the target organ after diagnosis of hypertension, and how often to evaluate it? When do patients need to start medication, how to adjust their lifestyle and behavior, and how to judge whether medication is effective? The above-mentioned contents can be transmitted to patients with high blood pressure with the help of medical professionals.

Last but not least, tertiary prevention of hypertension should also be mentioned. The tertiary prevention of the disease is mainly symptomatic treatment. It includes prevention of complications and disability; provision of rehabilitation medical care for those who have lost their labor force or become disabled; promotion of their early recovery in physical and mental aspects; recovery of their labor force, being diseased without disability or being disabled but useful; and preservation of their ability to create economic value and social labor value. The tertiary prevention of hypertension is mainly to prevent complications of hypertensive patients (who have experienced heart and cerebrovascular diseases) to rescue patients with severe hypertension to provide rehabilitation and to improve the quality of life. In that case, we, as the medical professionals, can provide guidance for rehabilitation for patients who have already experienced complications of hypertension; help their families and patients get a correct understanding of the disease, and provide various supports both physically and psychologically; and guide them to actively recover and return to the original life track as soon as possible.

3.2. *Seeing a doctor*

Seeing a doctor is the second level of medical communication. Many patients don't know how to see a doctor. To give a simple example, we often see a patient make a number of specialist appointments when he or she is not feeling well, because he/she doesn't know which appropriate department he/she shall visit. In many famous Grade A tertiary hospitals, you can also see some patients who want to make a specialist appointment, but they don't know how to register; therefore, they can only purchase at a high price from a scalper.

In a broad sense, "seeing a doctor" refers to all aspects related to medical treatment, including the process, system, laws, regulations, and guidance related to medical treatment.

There is an example of seeking medical service in other places below. A patient with a certain disease could not obtain the best treatment in a small local hospital. He decided to go to a big city for treatment, which is seeking medical service in other places. In this case, first of all, the patient needs to know which hospital he shall go to, and which hospital has the highest ranking in this specialty. Is the result of a search on a search engine reliable? Everyone knows that search results obtained through search engines are not reliable, such as the famous Wei Zexi incident: his choice of an inappropriate hospital (by searching on a search engine) caused his condition to deteriorate and his death. This is a typical example of loss of both life and property. Therefore, how do you choose an appropriate hospital and specialist? As medical communication professionals, we shall scientifically tell you the rankings of famous hospitals and specialists in the country. So, everyone knows which hospitals and specialists shall be selected after suffering from certain diseases. For example, the Hospital Management Institute, Fudan University publishes the rankings of famous hospitals and specialists in the country every year. This is a very professional and reliable ranking. Therefore, when we conduct a hospital introduction as medical professionals, we shall recommend or quote the rankings published by such formal institutions, and shall not recommend the search results obtained from search engines.

After learning which hospital he shall go to, the patient comes to the hospital, but he doesn't know how to register in the hospital. The specialist appointments have been fully booked, so he could only go to the emergency department. As everyone knows, the emergency department is to receive critically ill patients. However, the condition of the patient is complicated but not critical. First, the patient may need to queue for a long time. Second, there are many examinations and treatments that are unavailable in the emergency department. Therefore, the medical procedure of the patient has problems. At this time, what the patient urgently needs to know about is which diseases shall be seen in the emergency department, which diseases shall be seen in the clinic, and how to make an appointment online or by phone for specialist outpatient service. Through the above-mentioned science popularization, the patient learned that he shall go to a specialist clinic in a certain department, and booked the specialist outpatient service via the WeChat platform.

At the specialist clinic, the patient received careful diagnosis and treatment from an expert. The expert believed that the patient shall undergo further examination and treatment, preferably hospitalization. In this case, this is seeking medical service in other places. The patient is the insurance participant of medical insurance, but in other places, the patient does not know how to apply his medical insurance, including how to pay his medical expenses and how to apply for reimbursement. At present, the popularized medical knowledge he most needs is how to carry out the settlement of medical insurance in different places. Through the medical science popularization of how to settle medical insurance in different places, he learned about the policies related to medical insurance, roughly understood the medical expenses he needed to bear, and became more confident in treatment.

At the level of seeing a doctor, there is still much to be done in medical science popularization. For instance, how to call 120 emergency calls. Take Shanghai as an example. There are two types of 120 telephones in Shanghai. For non-emergency patients, such as those who need to be discharged from a hospital to a rehabilitation hospital, an old people's home, a nursing home, or their home, please just call 962120 and make an appointment. For critically ill patients, please call 120. The medical science popularization of different 120 emergency calls can help people occupy the first-aid 120 resources as little as possible, so that patients who need the most first-aid resources can get assistance first. In real life, there will be some patients or family members who provide the wrong address and contact information when dialing 120, so that first-aid personnel cannot reach the scene immediately, wasting the golden rescue time. Therefore, how to dial 120 correctly, and how to enable first-aid personnel to get the clearest instructions, also requires professional medical personnel to conduct medical science popularization.

3.3. *Opinions on disease*

Opinions on disease represent the third level of medical communication and the most difficult or most overlooked level. Attitude toward disease is more about medical humanities.

As a science, medicine has developed into the era of big data and artificial intelligence, but there are still many diseases that cannot be cured. As the famous American doctor E. L. Trudeau said, "To Cure Sometimes, To Relieve Often, To Comfort Always", and for many diseases, what doctors can do is to help and comfort.

However, many people have not yet been able to correctly understand the disease. They always believe that any disease can be cured if they go to the hospital to see a doctor. The value of medical communication with the level of attitude toward disease is helping people to treat diseases correctly and rationally, recognize the limitations of medicine, understand the natural laws of life and death, and choose the most appropriate treatment in the face of disease.

For example, for some patients with end-stage diseases, there are various tubes on their body to sustain life: a stomach tube, an evacuating catheter, a trachea cannula, etc. We can imagine this is very painful. Patients or their families are psychologically unable to accept the reality of their imminent death, or have considerable fear and anxiety about their death. Medical communication shall spread scientific knowledge about humanistic care for end-stage patients and their families, helping them to face disease and death of the patients rationally.

For patients with a survival period of less than six months, there is a medical philosophy called hospice care. Its essence is to provide patients with all aspects of care, supplemented by appropriate hospital or family medical care and nursing, to help them to reduce physical and mental pain, improve the quality of life, and help them calmly go through the final stages of life. However, at present, there are still many people who do not understand or accept this concept. Medical communication can spread and popularize this concept well, helping the public to understand who is suitable for hospice care and how to do it, so that everyone can be born smoothly and die peacefully.

In real life, there is still "hypochondriasis", which means that some people regard some common diseases as "dreadful monsters". The most common is depression. Realistically, everyone may experience a period of depressed mood, called depressive state, and if there is a significant and persistent depressed mood, it may be depression. WHO (World Health Organization) has listed depression as the fourth leading disease in the world, indicating that the incidence of depression is quite high. Many people who do not understand depression consider depression as a mental illness. There are also other people who think that people with depression are the ones who make a fuss about an imaginary illness. Actually, depression is a common mental illness. It can also be regarded as a chronic disease, which requires people to have a correct understanding of it. Many people do not understand why someone who seems to be cheerful is a patient with depression, and why a person who always wears a smile would choose to commit suicide. Ordinary people's misunderstanding of depression is the reason why many patients are unwilling to tell their illness. People with depression are afraid of being accused of making a fuss about an imaginary illness. Because they are the only ones who have depression around, they feel ashamed and shameful, and even think that it is their fault to get sick. Therefore, many people with depression choose not to receive treatment. In China, more than 70% of patients with depression have not been treated in a timely manner. They choose to ignore depression and their condition becomes more and more serious. For people with depression, perhaps, the best treatment is to accompany them to go through the depression period. Therefore, in the field of medical communication, it is essential for us to conduct medical science popularization constantly, so as to help people correctly understand diseases such as depression, identify and help people with depression in a timely manner, and understand how to accompany and take care of them.

Chapter 10

Science Popularization Principles and Skills of Doctors, Nurses, and Technicians

1. The principle of popularization of science for medical personnel

1.1. *Principle of accessibility*

The word "plain to understand" comes from Deng Xiaoping's "the situation of victory in the leap to the central plains and future policies and strategies": "These sixteen words are plain to understand". It means that the general public can understand. It also means simple and clear.

The first principle of medical science is to be easy to understand. Why does it have to be easy to understand? Medicine is a subject of science, but also more esoteric. Generally speaking, a medical student must go through many years of training to master certain medical professional knowledge. Teaching professional medical knowledge to the ordinary people not only requires a lot of time and energy, but also requires the general public to have a high level of knowledge base. However, ordinary people have no need to become doctors; there is no need to spend a lot of time to master the professional medical knowledge, and they just need to know the basic medical knowledge. So for the ordinary people, if you talk about medical science at a professional level, that is to say, if you use professional terms and medical jargons to explain medicine, the public would have no interest to read or understand. Science popularization means to introduce medical knowledge to the general public in a simple and easily understood way. Therefore, it is necessary to follow the basic knowledge level of the general public and try to explain medical phenomena and medical problems in an easy and understandable way.

Let's analyze these from several forms of medical science popularization. Medical science articles are written for the public to read. They must be narrated and introduced in the popular language that the public like and understand, so that the public can understand and accept them. If the whole article is a textbook style of boring introduction, including a lot of technical terms, medical terms, English symbols, the reader will get "a headache" and feel "bored". How can they like this medical science article? Therefore, to enhance the readability of medical science articles, the key is to try to make the highly professional medical knowledge easy to understand and make the boring and dull introduction vivid and interesting. Let's look at a simple example. Cerebral infarction is a very common disease. "Cerebral infarction is defined as localized ischemic necrosis or softening of brain tissue due to impaired blood supply to the brain, ischemia, or hypoxia", one article said. This statement is profound and it is easy for medical professionals to understand it, but for the non-medical general public, they cannot understand it, so they have no interest in reading the rest of this article. "Cerebral infarction is a type of stroke caused by a blockage of blood vessels in the brain". Compared to the previous article, the statement of this article explains cerebral infarction in a relatively simple and understandable way, so that the ordinary people can understand it and are willing to read on.

This not only applies to medical science articles, but also other forms of science articles. For example, as mentioned in the previous chapter, Alzheimer's disease is now very common. But the terminology is such that the public doesn't know what the disease is and won't care. There's actually another name for Alzheimer's disease in Chinese called senile dementia. If this relatively simple word is used to describe the disease, then even the general public with average knowledge can understand what it is. Also innovative ways, such as the form of cross talk to explain the disease, will have a good dissemination effect.

For the promotion of popular new media and we media, being easy to understand is also an important principle. Although the readers surfing the Internet include a part of the population with medical knowledge, most are still at a basic level of knowledge; so it's still about the needs of the masses. Popularizing science is like cooking a dish. Medical knowledge is like an enormous raw material. It needs to be processed and integrated, just like chopping vegetables and stir-frying vegetables. With the right taste, try to fit the taste of the public. If you put a bunch of raw materials on the table, nobody wants to eat them. The raw material is like a professional medical academic paper, which is not understood by non-professionals. Of course, other ingredients should not be added in order to pursue the taste. This is alarmist, which should be put an end to. If we directly put a medical paper in the new media and we media, the public will not read it, and medical professionals will not read it in these media, because there are other ways to access the medical paper such as through searching a special database, then the audience of this article will be very rare. For example, we published an article on medical science in new media: "on standardized diagnosis, treatment process and progress of ischemic stroke". Such an article, with such a professional title, would not be of interest to most ordinary people. Instead, if it is replaced with a popular science article: "How do you tell if you're having a stroke?" Such easy-to-understand, concise and clear title will attract ordinary people to continue to read, so it can play the purpose of the popularization and dissemination of medical knowledge.

1.2. *"With the help of a hot spot" principle*

This is the age of scarcity. We can see a lot of information, but notice very little. There's less information that we can talk about as a topic. Information is abundant and attention resources are limited. So, we always pay attention to the hot news first, and we are always attracted by the hot topics that take away our attention. "With the help of a hot spot" is a common way to attract attention. Hot topics attract a lot of attention and many people will watch and participate in the discussion. In the short term, attention is drawn to one or two hot topics and other important and interesting information is ignored. In other words, we automatically filter out other information. If some product information happens to appear in the hot spot, the product will become the focus of word-of-mouth talkers. After watching the excitement, people may seriously consider whether to buy the products of that brand. The same is true in health care. If health-related information happens to appear in hot spots, it will become the focus of people's discussion. After watching the buzz, people may seriously consider adopting the advice in the health-related message.

Generally speaking, hot spots can be divided into two types: One is predictable hot spots, such as various holidays and so on; the other is unpredictable hot spots, such as emergencies.

When it comes to emergencies, let's look at some examples. As we all know, earthquake is a disastrous event; once there is a big earthquake, it will cause great harm. Earthquake, also known as ground motion, ground vibration, is the crust in the process of rapid release of energy caused by vibration, a natural phenomenon that produces seismic waves. The main cause of earthquakes is the collision between the tectonic plates and the edges of the plates. Earthquakes often cause serious casualties, fire, flood, toxic gas leakage, spread of bacteria and radioactive materials, and may also cause tsunami, landslide, collapse, cracks, and other secondary disasters.

According to statistics, there are more than 5 million earthquakes on earth every year, that is, there are tens of thousands of earthquakes every day. Most of them are too small or too far away to be felt. There are about ten or twenty earthquakes that can cause serious harm to human beings. There are about one or two earthquakes that can cause particularly severe damage. The current level of technology is not able to predict the arrival of earthquakes, and for a long time in the future, the earthquake is also unpredictable. Examples of successful earthquake prediction are largely coincidental. For earthquakes, what we should do is to improve the seismic level of the building and prepare for good defense, rather than predicting the earthquake.

Japan is a country prone to earthquakes. The Japanese islands lie at the boundary between the Pacific plate, the Philippine sea plate, the Eurasian plate, and the north American continental plate. According to tectonic plate theory, the Pacific plate is thinner, denser, and lower in position. When the Pacific plate moves horizontally westward, it dives beneath the adjacent Eurasian plate. Therefore, when the Eurasian plate and the Pacific plate collide and squeeze, the rock layers at the junction of the two plates will deform and break, resulting in volcanic eruptions and earthquakes. As a volcanic country, earthquakes are common in Japan, and people feel them almost every day. So what happened after the earthquake in Japan? At 7:58 am on June 19, 2018, a magnitude 6 earthquake struck Osaka, Japan. According to statistics, 30 hours after the earthquake, a total of 4 people died and 376 were injured. The earthquake affected traffic, buildings, and public facilities. The earthquake happened in the morning, during the rush hour, and many people were trapped on the way. Subway and light rail lines were also largely out of service. The conductor and the police stood at a distance of ten paces along the route to guide the passengers to evacuate in an orderly manner. The station also opened a wire fence nearby to help evacuees to get off the line as quickly as possible. Evacuees walked along the line to nearby stations without jumping in line, without crowding, as if nothing had happened. The railway company released the latest train operation information through the bulletin board and the Internet to help to evacuate the stranded people at the station as soon as possible. The Osaka government was the first to open 391 shelters for the homeless. The earthquake left many store shelves scattered and unable to open. In the few regular convenience stores and restaurants, water and food were offered to the refugees at a discount. Although the shelves of drinking water and food were almost empty, people only took basic necessities without looting. In addition to some railway and water gas line facilities to be repaired, within 24 hours after the earthquake, Osaka urban traffic has been partially normal, part of the subway, aircraft and other external means of transportation have been restored, casualties are also within the controllable range, and there is no major secondary disaster.

As we know, earthquakes cannot be accurately predicted with current scientific and technological means. Once a major earthquake occurs, the human and economic damage will be immeasurable. From Japan's successful experience in dealing with earthquake, we can see that there is a lot of science that can be done about earthquake, and a lot can be done as a normal situation, rather than an isolated emergency. For the medical science about earthquake, what we can do is to save ourselves or others when the earthquake comes. How to protect yourself and others when earthquake causes fire, flood, poisonous gas leakage, bacteria and radioactive material diffusion, and possibly also tsunami, landslide, collapse, cracks in the ground, and other secondary disasters? In an earthquake, how to follow a certain order and avoid the occurrence of stampede? If there is a stampede, how to carry out first aid and so on. Such science popularization and publicity topics should be carried out as a routine in an area and country with a high incidence of earthquakes. This can avoid getting into a panic when the earthquake comes.

Of course, when the earthquake occurs as an emergency, it is still necessary to strengthen some medical science education for the public. For example, the old saying "after a major disaster, there must be a pandemic" means that infectious diseases may appear after a major disaster. So after the earthquake, topics such as how to prevent infectious diseases and what symptoms to look out for and other medical knowledge will have a good effect. However, after the occurrence of earthquake as an emergency, as a sudden hot spot, various contents related to earthquake, including medical knowledge, will receive a lot of attention in a short time. At this time, the popularization of science can also play a wider and more effective dissemination role than usual. For example, after an earthquake, topics such as cardiopulmonary resuscitation and the handling of the seriously injured may receive more than the normal level of search volume and attention.

We are glad to see that when various disasters come, the popularization of medical science on how to save people has been valued by the medical profession, and relevant attempts have been made. Published by the People's Medical Publishing House, *Pictures of Disaster Escape and Rescue Science Series* is the first science popularization series of disaster escape and rescue in the form of cartoon. It is easy to understand and vivid. It has not only been well received and welcomed by the people, but also won the second prize of National Science and Technology Progress Award in 2018.

When it comes to predictable hot spots, it's common to see them on regular holidays. For example, the Spring Festival is the most important festival for Chinese people. Every year, the Spring Festival is a time for family reunion and dinner. The New Year's eve dinner is the most important meal of the year. People pay great attention to the "New Year's eve dinner". In addition to family reunion, people also pray for the health and safety of the family. The reunion dinner is the highlight of the Spring Festival. It is not only rich and diverse, but also has many traditions. During the Spring Festival holiday, a lot of people will eat and drink, and therefore, every year before and after the Spring Festival, the number of gastrointestinal discomfort patients, diabetic patients, pancreatitis patients will increase. In view of this phenomenon, the popularization of science on how to have a reasonable diet and how to control blood sugar for diabetic patients before and after the Spring Festival each year will be a typical hot spot of the Spring Festival, and it will also receive unexpected effects.

1.3. *"Appeals to humor" principle*

The word "幽默" (*youmo*) is a transliteration of the English word "Humor". It means something funny or being funny. It was Lin Yutang, a master of Chinese sinology, who first introduced the word to China. This is a word with both pronunciation and meaning, and its expression is just right.

"There are broad and narrow senses of humor. In English usage, it often includes vulgar jokes..." In the narrow sense, humor is different from sarcasm and ridicule, which all contain the meaning of "laugh". However, "laugh" also includes wry smile, guffaw smile, weak smile, silly smile, that is to say, the meaning and attitude of laughter are different. Some "laugh" is sour and spicy, some "smile" is kind, some "laugh" is contemptuous, some "laugh" is sympathy, some "laugh" is based on the whole outlook on life, some "laugh" is the sustenance of thought. The best humor, of course, is to show "the brilliance of the soul and the richness of wisdom... Of all the styles, humor is the most emotional" (Lin Yutang, *On Reading and Humor*, published by Contemporary World Publishing House). Humor is a kind of wisdom that can arouse some emotion in human psychology, and some kind of processing or destruction of reality after proper regulation of logic. Humor or funny has been elevated to the realm of philosophical research; it is no exaggeration to say that humor is a philosophy. Humor often brings joy to people. It is characterized by wit, self-mockery, ridicule, fun, and so on. Indeed, humor helps to remove hostility, ease friction, and prevent escalation. Others believe humor can boost morale and productivity. A Colorado company found that mid-level executives who took humor classes increased productivity by 15% over nine months, while the number of sick days dropped by half.

Humor is actually an evolution of language. When the same meaning is expressed in different ways, it may feel completely different to the recipient. China has thousands of years of civilization; language and culture gradually mature. Language has a gradual process from primitive to evolutionary. For example, when people first said "shit" or "pee", they didn't say it directly. Instead, they said "go to the outhouse" or "go to the toilet". Later, they said "go to the bathroom" or "go to the dressing room". This is the result of the evolution of language due to the increasing complexity of human relations and the progress of civilization. As the saying goes, practice makes perfect, so do words, especially between jokes. For example, when someone says, "I have enough to eat, then the whole family is not hungry", what we hear is: This person is living alone. The writer Mark Twain once said: "quitting smoking is the easiest, I quit more than two hundred times". People will understand: he has not given up! The meaning of this statement is clear, and it is very funny. It is obviously an artistic grammar. It is a creative language. That's humor. A writer with a sense of humor can make his works interesting. A good sense of humor in an orator keeps the audience laughing. Entrepreneurs have a sense of humor that makes subordinates feel friendly. Educators with a sense of humor will be more effective in enlightening the mind of the recipient; A sense of humor in a marriage can make ordinary life happy and warm.

There are nine benefits of humor: humor reduces stress, helps communication, overcomes fear, makes people comfortable, relaxed people, relieves pain, boosts the immune system, fosters optimism, and spreads happiness. Humor in life can increase the fun and intimacy of words, and using humor in medical science popularization and communication is easier to gain public support and public recognition than mechanically copying and preaching.

Let's look at some examples. "Coolest Ethnic" is a popular song sung by Phoenix Legend, which is known to the public because of its catchy melody. "Coolest Ethnic" won the title of "Baidu Music TOP500 Songs" for 27 weeks and was also elected as the champion of "Baidu Music Top 10 Songs of 2012" and "the most popular song of the year of the 11th CCTV-MV music grand ceremony in 2012". Its arrangement is relaxed and cheerful, melody is very dynamic, and the lyrics are very close to life. This song has a broad mass base; when you walk in the street, you can hear the melody of this song everywhere. In May 2017, Dr. Bing from the Department of Thoracic Surgery of Peking Union Medical College Hospital changed his music video "Coolest First-Aid" with the tune of "Coolest Ethnic". The video has been viewed more than 1.4 million times and received more than 10,000 likes in just half a day. With funny painting style and fluent speech, Dr. Bing teaches the first-aid techniques for cardiopulmonary resuscitation (CPR). Someone said: "learned knowledge, crazy ears, blind eyes!" For the general public, learning CPR skills is necessary, but learning CPR skills is also very boring. Boring learning content will make people feel boring, so the learning effect and motivation will be reduced, and the goal of learning cannot be achieved. However, through such humorous and interesting video, the public can learn how to perform cardiopulmonary resuscitation very easily. In a pleasant and cheerful atmosphere, the knowledge of cardiopulmonary resuscitation is unconsciously increased, and the public may also increase their interest in the knowledge of cardiopulmonary resuscitation, so as to further understand and master it.

For example, there is a popular German children's medical science book *The Adventure of Bacteria in the Human Body*. It's about a little bacterial monster that embarks on a human adventure that starts in the human mouth and continues down the nose, throat and blood vessels, lungs, and stomach until food is eventually digested and absorbed in the gut. This is a popular science book that parents and children can read together, with graphic pictures. It is not only funny and easy to read, but also lets the children know about human body and medical knowledge, and teaches the children that diarrhea is not annoying, vomiting is good for the body, and the thick liquid in the intestinal tract is kind and lovely. Such humorous and interesting science books will be very popular with children, including parents. For adults, too, the more humorous and interesting the medical story, the more deeply rooted it is.

The above three common principles in medical science are the basic principles that every medical professional should master. Of course, there are many other skills and means to do medical science, which can be improved through learning and understanding.

2. How to write medical science articles

Medical science articles are the most common way of medical communication. It can be published in newspapers and magazines, and it can also appear in the popular new media forms such as microblog and WeChat. For medical science articles, first of all, the content must be accurate, which means that the author, that is, the medical staff must consult the relevant literature and materials. Secondly, the content should be closely related to the current hot issues of public concern. During flu season, for example, there are a lot of science articles on flu types. For science articles, there is also a very important point, which is to pay attention to timeliness. Last summer, a pregnant woman jumped from a building in Yulin, Shaanxi province. Combined with this tragic event, a lot can be done, especially about the rights of pregnant women and their mothers. If you do it in the period of public attention, you will get the best results. If you do science popularization after the period of public attention, your results will decrease.

Medical science articles, in addition to the science of related diseases, also can cover some medical-related laws and regulations of science. For example, the science about organ donation. The general public's lack of medical knowledge is not only in the diseases, but also in medical-related laws and regulations, which need to be spread and popularized.

In today's society, the doctor–patient relationship is quite tense. So medical communication and popular science can also make some efforts on how to improve the doctor–patient relationship, which is also helpful to build a harmonious doctor–patient relationship.

In China, humanistic care for patients is not enough. Humanistic care for patients is also a good entry point for medical science articles. For example, by telling patients what "patient satisfaction" is, it explains to the patient how the professional organization rates the patient satisfaction of the hospital. This can help patients to clarify their questions about the investigation.

With the development of medicine today, more and more attention has been paid to the prevention of diseases. As an ancient Chinese saying goes, "a good doctor treats diseases that have not yet happened". Therefore, many medical science articles will not only talk about the disease itself, but also pay more attention to the prevention of the disease.

In short, the scope of medical science articles can be very wide. However, the article should not only meet the needs of patients, but also be concise and focused on timeliness, so as to achieve a better communication effect. With the development of society and the transformation of medical model, medical science popularization in the new period should not only inherit the characteristics of traditional medical science popularization, but also explore the new situation, new content, new problems, and the new characteristics of medical science popularization. Accordingly, it also has a higher requirement of medical science creators.

3. How to make contact with traditional media

The word "media" comes from the Latin word "Medius", transliterated as the medium, which means between the two. Media is the medium that transmits information. It refers to a tool, channel, carrier, intermediary, or technical means that people use to convey information and obtain information. The media can also be thought of as all the technical means by which information is transmitted from the source to the trusted. Media has two meanings. One is the object that carries information, and the other is the entity that information can be stored, presented, processed, and transmitted.

Compared with the emerging network media in recent years, traditional mass communication means that the media regularly release information to the public or provide education and entertainment platform through some mechanical device, mainly including newspapers, outdoor, communication, radio, television, and other network media in the traditional sense.

Although various network media prevail, traditional media still have a certain status. Some people, such as the elderly in remote areas with underdeveloped Internet connection, still rely on newspapers, TV, and other traditional media for information.

So how do medical communicators make contact with traditional media?

3.1. *Newspapers*

Newspapers are printed on paper, and generally have a large circulation and a fast frequency. Many newspapers are published every day and have a fixed number of readers. Different newspapers may have different styles and target different people. Many newspapers have special sections on medicine and health, and some have sections on science. When doing medical communication, it is mainly carried out in these two sections. There are usually reporters and editors of newspaper columns. For ordinary writers, they can pay attention to the contents of the medical and health or science column of the newspaper, and then choose the medical field they are good at and write about medical communication for submission. Of course, when submitting articles, remember to be short, concise, easy to understand, and readable, so that the contribution rate will be relatively high, because in the era of fast food culture, no one will take the time to read a long article. For more famous medical experts or science experts, the reporter may make an interview and write a news report. In this case, the authors are journalists, not medical experts or science specialists themselves. Therefore, we should pay attention to the communication process with journalists to ensure that the journalists' understanding of medical knowledge is correct and the medical content written by the journalists is not biased. Otherwise, it may lead to ambiguity or misunderstanding of readers, and also violates the concept of medical communication to disseminate correct medical knowledge.

3.2. *Magazine*

Magazines are also traditional media. The magazine printing is more exquisite than the newspaper, and generally has a specific target population, but the publication cycle is relatively long: some need a week, some need a month. Not all magazines are good for medical communication. Health and wellness magazines are better for medical communication than fashion magazines. Magazines, like newspapers, have reporters and editors. Medical science articles written in magazines need pictures and words to be vivid and interesting. As the space in the magazine is more extensive, they can better highlight the topics to be propagated, but they need to be more careful to ensure the accuracy and reliability of the contents. For some famous medical experts, the magazine will ask for an invited article or make an interview; the difference is that the former content is written by the medical experts themselves, while the latter is written by journalists. As mentioned above, if it is written by a journalist, the journalist must confirm the contents without any ambiguity or misunderstanding.

3.3. *TV*

As a traditional media platform, the television's biggest difference from newspapers and magazines is that it is three-dimensional, with visual and auditory impact, that is, with the sense of scene and intuitive feelings. Although many young people have started to widely use new media and we media, TV is still a very popular traditional media. There are many programs about health, health preservation, and medical treatment on TV, which are also popular with the audience. Every network may have several typical health and wellness programs. For this kind of programs, first of all, its audience will be very wide: people who have a TV at home can view the program, its coverage is big and there is no threshold. Secondly, the introduction of health or healthy habits by TV can be more intuitively understood by the audience and more easily accepted. However, we need to be clear that such programs are not advertisements and should not be used for certain companies or products. We should also follow some principles when conducting medical science communication on TV. Considering the different educational levels of the audience, the content should be as simple and understandable as possible, which means that ordinary people can understand it. Don't use technical and complicated terms. Secondly, the forms of popular science can be vivid and interesting, such as sitcoms, sketches or storytelling. Don't be confined to the form of lectures, and don't make such programs into academic reports, so that the audience will not be interested. When making popular science program, the producers and hosts should communicate well in advance. Since each program will have a certain theme, producers and hosts will also have certain requirements. They can cooperate on the basis of the accuracy of the content, and remember that the interviewee cannot ramble on television, or arbitrarily exaggerate the effect of one treatment or belittle the effect of other treatments; the content must be scientific, then universal.

3.4. *Radio*

Radio transmits content through sound. There are a lot of programs on modern radio that are interview programs or health care programs. Unlike television, newspapers, and magazines, radio can only be listened to, not seen. Compared with television, the audience of radio has gradually declined. People who still use radio in modern life are rare, and it is probably only in remote areas or among the elderly who still listen to radio. But there are some benefits. For example, you can listen to it anytime and anywhere, just like you can't watch TV while driving, but you can listen to the radio. Listen to it while you're resting or taking a nap. Although the radio is almost nowhere to be found, there are all kinds of software to listen to it. The easiest way is to listen to it on a mobile phone, and for those with vision problems or visual fatigue, radio can be a good tool. Since radio programs are the art of hearing, it is important to select those with standard pronunciation and relatively good timbre for science popularization or dissemination. Imagine, if a medical worker's pronunciation is not standard, sometimes with some local accent, it is not only unpleasant, but also may cause the audience to misunderstand the meaning, which is very bad for medical communication. Radio programs usually have hosts. Before making the program, the hosts and interviewees should have some communication and make some attempts on the basis of ensuring the accuracy and reliability of the transmitted content. You can tell stories and give examples to impress your audience.

4. How to control the public opinion of the epidemic situation

Epidemic situation is the occurrence of epidemics and the spread of diseases, that is, the occurrence and spread of infectious diseases. Here's an example to help you to understand. The SARS epidemic in 2003 was a typical infectious disease, and its occurrence and spread were epidemic cases. The SARS epidemic in that year was quite serious.

Public opinion refers to the social attitude generated and held by the people as the subject to social managers, enterprises, individuals, and other organizations as well as their political, social, and moral orientations regarding the occurrence, development, and change of intermediary social events in a certain social space. It is the sum total of the beliefs, attitudes, opinions and emotions expressed by the larger masses about various phenomena and problems in the society. As a society with highly developed information, people can learn more information through the Internet and express themselves freely through the Internet. Therefore, in modern society, the power of online public opinion cannot be ignored. Network public opinion is the mapping of social public opinion in the Internet space and the direct reflection of social public opinion. Traditional social public opinion is in the folk, existing in the public's ideas and opinions. The former is hard to catch, the latter is fleeting; the public opinion can only be obtained through public observation, secret visits, public opinion survey, and other methods. These methods are inefficient, with few samples and easy to be biased, and cost a lot. With the development of the Internet, the public often express their opinions in an information-based way. Network public opinions can be easily obtained by automatic network scraping and other technical means, with high efficiency and information fidelity (no artificial processing), with full coverage. The power of online public opinion is powerful. A small event can explode in a short period of time with the help of others. For example, not long ago, a video, in which a woman stood up for rights in a famous 4S shop of a car brand, was quickly spread on the Internet, and everyone commented on it. The problem of upholding rights, which had been unresolved for a long time, was quickly solved by this propagation. But at the same time, the woman's personal information has been released, and some people even doubt her character, causing great trouble to the woman. Therefore, network public opinion needs correct guidance, and its hidden power cannot be ignored.

Health authorities, such as the CDC, should regularly release surveillance reports that tell people about recent infectious disease surveillance. There can be a panic during an outbreak, especially during a major outbreak. The main reason is that people don't know the specific situation and don't know what to do, and then there is a huge panic. There are also some people who are malicious or make trouble or hope to attract others' attention. They like to spread some rumors on the Internet, such as how many people died of a certain disease in a certain place. As the speed of the Internet spread is hard to imagine, it is easy to cause people's panic.

In the event of an outbreak, the official health administration should release to the public the latest surveillance of the outbreak, and in the case of a major outbreak, it is better to publish it daily, so that people can clearly understand the specific situation and will not listen to the unreliable information. Secondly, the authorities should also tell people what to pay attention to when dealing with this kind of infectious disease, how to prevent it, what symptoms to look out for, where to go to see a doctor when the disease occurs, and so on. In this way, people can know how to face these diseases, have a better understanding, and there will be no widespread panic. The disclosure of information can minimize the occurrence of public opinion on the epidemic.

Of course, those who spread false information and malicious ideas should be banned on the Internet. When necessary, we can use legal means to punish those who spread rumors, and intensify the punishment on those who spread rumors, so that those who spread rumors will no longer dare to do so. In addition, strengthening the management of the Internet, finding the response of public opinion, timely reporting and sorting out, and releasing reliable information by the officials can effectively avoid the spread of rumors.

5. How to choose what to spread

When carrying out medical communication, the first problem is topic selection. What content can be spread, and what content is not suitable to spread?

This is different from the topic selection of scientific research papers. The topic selection of scientific research papers focuses on innovation, that is to say, it needs to be different from previous papers and be original. Medical communication subjects are more cautious, and the main criteria are scientific, accuracy, and practicality.

Being scientific means that the topic selection should be guided by scientific thought and based on facts. Here's a simple example. When doing the popularization of high blood pressure medicine, some professionals talk about "high salt diet can lead to high blood pressure". This topic is scientific, because the association between high salt diet and high blood pressure has been confirmed in large-scale clinical trials, which is based on evidence-based medicine, so it is a good choice. However, if he chooses the topic of "patients with high blood pressure can no longer eat salt", it is exaggerating and rambling, which violates the scientific principle and is inappropriate.

Accuracy is the degree to which an event is accurate. In medical communication, we pay special attention to accuracy because medical communication is aimed at ordinary people who have limited medical knowledge. If what we promote and advocate is wrong, or not widely proven, or controversial in its current state, it is likely to lead to ambiguity or misdirection in the general population, which could be harmful to health. For example, whether genetically modified food is beneficial or harmful to human body has been debated in the scientific community. For such controversial content, medical communication is not suitable for extensive dissemination and promotion. He Jiankui, for example, is one of *Nature* magazine's top 10 scientific figures in 2018. He got the attention because he created the world's first genetically edited babies. However, after making his work known, he was widely criticized for ignoring moral and ethical guidelines and exposing the babies to unknown risks for uncertain benefits. The inclusion in the top 10 figures is not a positive one, but a cautionary tale. It would be irresponsible to make Dr. He's scientific findings widely available as part of medical communication when they were controversial. In fact, some recent research results have not been widely confirmed and recognized, so it is best not to use them as topics of medical communication. Because these results may change after a period of time, with some of them being proved, and some of them disproved. If we promote and disseminate these results before they have been widely proved, it will violate the principle of accuracy of medical communication and may mislead or even harm the health of the people.

Practicality means that the content of medical communication should meet the practical needs of the masses, rather than being too esoteric or too rare. The target population of medical communication is the general population with general knowledge, not medical professionals, so if very esoteric or rare content is transmitted, the general population is not interested and cannot understand, then the significance of medical communication is lost. For example, a medical professional gives a popular science lecture, and the title is "the serum microRNA-4286 expression and the relationship with gastric cancer". This is a scientific research topic and looks like the title of a scientific paper; it is very suitable for communication at an academic conference or in academic journals, but it is not suitable for medical communication to the public. If replaced with "who needs regular screening for gastric cancer risk", this might be a more suitable topic for the public.

In terms of the selection criteria of medical communication, there are still some basic requirements. In the beginning of medical communication, medical professionals often choose some topics that are not suitable for communication, which results in the unpopular dissemination and promotion of the topic. Although the form is vivid and interesting, the content is not accurate or reliable, misleading the general public. Which topics are suitable for communication, and which are not, are what we need to know and make clear when we start medical communication in the first place.

Part V
Practice

Chapter 11

Medical Communication Practice — Taking "Da Yi Xiao Hu" Medical Communication Think Tank as an Example

"Da Yi Xiao Hu" Medical Communication Think Tank signifies "understanding general medical knowledge and knowing about family care". Guided by China Association for Science and Technology, the editorial committee comprises clinical experts from China Science Writers Association and Medical and Health Society of the Shanghai Science Writers Association. It is a nonprofit brand that integrates talent training, original works, we media operation, offline programs, science popularization practice, and research. It is also a key project of the Shanghai Science and Technology Committee and Shanghai Association for Science and Technology.

The five key characteristics of "Da Yi Xiao Hu" are as follows:

(1) Authoritativeness. The editorial team is composed of hundreds of first-line clinical experts and health communication specialists from nationwide, among which three clinical experts are winners of the State Science and Technology Advancement Award.
(2) Academic attribute. All the works are not only based on the western medicine theory but also include the science popularization knowledge of traditional Chinese medicine, which lays great emphasis on "prevention before a disease arises, preventing disease from exacerbating". This

integration of the Chinese and Western medicine reflects its feature of academic attribute and also is close to daily life.

(3) Public good. Medical professionals volunteer to perform the editorial and background operations without involving commercial activities.

(4) Originality. All the science popularization works are created by the editorial team to ensure the authenticity. This prevents errors due to plagiarism on the internet.

(5) Diversity of content forms and broadness of communication. Various types of science popularization works are presented on this platform, including cartoons, crosstalk, songs, body painting, microfilms, poetry, and short plays. Also, with the characteristic of new media such as fast dissemination, wide range, abundant amount of information, and strong interaction, science popularization works could be extensively spread via this platform.

1. The construction of "Da Yi Xiao Hu" medical communication think tank

1.1. *About "Da Yi Xiao Hu" team (Table 11.1)*

Dr. Wang Tao, the team founder and Editor-in-Chief, is Executive Deputy Director of Emergency Department, Director of Emergency Management Office, and the Director of Disaster Medicine Education Division from Shanghai East Hospital affiliated to Tongji University. He is the Director of the Health and Medical Communication Research Center, the School of Media and Communication, Shanghai Jiao Tong University, and Chairman of Medical Popularization Society of the China Science Writers Association. His awards include Shanghai Science Popularization Outstanding Person Award which is the highest rank of Shanghai Popular Science Education Innovation Awards, China Science and Technology Communication Award, and Top Ten Science Communicators from the China Association for Science and Technology. He also received the first prize of Shanghai Science and Technology Advancement Award, Popular Science Award of the Chinese Medical Science and Technology Award, Gold Prize for Outstanding Popular Science Works from China Science Writers Association, and National Excellent Popular Science Works from Ministry of Science and Technology of China.

Table 11.1 List of some "Da Yi Xiao Hu" team members.

Adviser	Qian Xuhong	"973" Chief Scientist Academician of the Chinese Academy of Engineering Director of Shanghai Science Writers Association
Adviser	Jiang Shiliang	Senior Editor of Wen Wei Po Executive Deputy Director and Secretary-General of Shanghai Science Writers Association Executive member of the China Science Writers Association
Adviser	Wang Lixiang	Director of Emergency Medical Center, China Armed Police Corps Hospital Chairman of Popular Science Branch, Chinese Medical Association Chairman of Cardiopulmonary Resuscitation Society, Chinese Research Hospital Association
Adviser	Guo Shubin	Director of Emergency Department, Beijing Chaoyang Hospital Chairman designate of Popular Science Branch, Chinese Medical Association President of Popular Science Branch, Chinese Medical Doctor Association
Honorary Editor-in-Chief	Fang Binghua	Gold Prize Winner of Outstanding Popular Science Works, China Science Writers Association Vice President of Shanghai Medical Ethics Committee Deputy Party secretary of Shanghai Shen Kang Hospital Development Center
Honorary Editor-in-Chief	Tang Qin	Director of Science and Technology Popularization Division, Chinese Medical Association
Editor-in-Chief	Wang Tao	Executive Deputy Director of Emergency Department, Shanghai East Hospital affiliated to Tongji University Chairman of Medical Popularization Society, China Science Writers Association Chairman of Cardiopulmonary Resuscitation Branch, Chinese Medical Doctor Association

(Continued)

Table 11.1   (*Continued*)

Editor-in-Chief	Dong Jian	Winner of the State Science and Technology Advancement Award Shanghai Leading Talents Director of Orthopedics Department, Zhongshan Hospital, Fudan University
Executive Chief Editor	Sun Feng	Vice Director of Emergency and Outpatient Department, Shanghai Putuo People's Hospital
Deputy Director of the Chief Editor's Office	Mou Yi	Professor of the School of Media and Communication, Shanghai Jiao Tong University
Assistant to the Editor-in-Chief	Jiang Ping	Assistant Professor, Laboratory of Biochemical Pharmacology, Shanghai Mental Health Center Program Leader of Da Yi Xiao Hu — Yellow Bracelets Home (science popularization for Alzheimer's disease)
Assistant to the Editor-in-Chief	Ma Lulu	Publicity Section, Shanghai Putuo District Central Hospital
Assistant to the Editor-in-Chief	Han Rui	Attending Physician, Shanghai Huadong Hospital, Fudan University

Dr. Dong Jian, Editor-in-Chief, is the Director of Orthopedics Department of Zhongshan Hospital, Fudan University. He is the recipient of the State Science and Technology Advancement Award.

Based on the Healthy China 2030 Strategic Plan, there are 92 online columns and 20 launched programs. The team has produced more than 500 original works and achieved over 200 million views online annually. There are more than 50,000 participants attending theme activities. Team members are all medical professionals who run operations of the communication platforms in their spare time aiming to ensure the authoritative, scientific, objective, and public wellness nature. Science popularization works are all original works including articles, cartoons, songs, and videos.

1.2. Scientific popularization creation

There are 92 online columns in the "Da Yi Xiao Hu" Medical Communication Think Tank. It also provides online nursing consultation.

Most of the editors in charge of each column or program come from the clinical front line. The content of popular science covers all aspects of healthcare. In addition to internal medicine, surgery, obstetrics and gynecology, and pediatrics, it includes the information about public health, disease control and prevention, advanced and pre-hospital first aid, tips for doctor visit, rehabilitation and nursing, medication safety, interpretation of lab test, community health service, general practice, hospital management, health insurance system, interpretation of healthcare policies, and media communication of medical popularization. "Da Yi Xiao Hu" also involves the research hotspots or frontier disciplines such as the integration of traditional Chinese and Western medicine, medical humanities, medical ethics, medical communication, behavioral medicine, plateau diseases, and so on. It provides timely and useful medical popularization for the public by focusing on healthcare industry hotspots and performing a comprehensive and deep-dive analysis.

Medical popularization works include articles, cartoons, songs, body painting, crosstalk, short plays, videos, and microfilms. There have been nearly 600 original works and over 200 million views have been achieved online. The most popular works are about medical specialties, prevention and treatment of conditions, rehabilitation, and nursing which are also key contents on the WeChat official accounts platform. Over 30 columns are set up follow those different directions of medical popularization works. For internal medicine, there are columns such as "Achieve Internal Health", "Thriving Heart" "Stepping on 'Blood' without Trace", "Everlasting Kidney", "Kidney and Heart", "Pancreas and Sepsis". For surgery, there are columns of "Pursuing Healthy Spine", "Talk About Bone and Muscle", "Urology and Reproduction", "Peaceful Gut", "Eyeopening", and "Anesthesia and Medical Popularization". In terms of obstetrics and gynecology and pediatrics, there are "Xiami Mummy", "Woman Flowers", "Preemie Angels", and "Raising Cute Baby". Other columns include "Nutrition and Health", "Skin Beauty Solutions", "Go Up in Smoke", "Acupuncture and Health", "Pain-free", "Bone Health", "Inspiration", "Psychological topics", as well as "Tips for a Successful Doctor Visit", "Health Insurance Policy", "Patient–physician communication", and so on. Online nursing consultation is one program on the "Da Yi Xiao Hu" WeChat official account. It provides nursing consultation on rehabilitation and care in a fixed period of weekdays.

The team focuses on the innovation of new media use. For instance, medical professionals write, direct, and perform themselves in a way of traditional science popularization in order to extend the duration and space of medical service. There are various types of science popularization works on the WeChat office account. Apart from the traditional articles, there have been popular science comics, readings, cross talks, songs, body paintings, microfilms, poetries, and short plays. The short play and microfilms produced by the team won the first prize in the Shanghai Medical Association Youth Competition on Science Popularization, and the "Best Director Award" in the Jury Prize of the 2017 Shanghai International Popular Science MicroFilm Competition.

1.3. *Launch the scientific popularization programs*

The team has launched 20 science popularization programs that realized online communication to offline face-to-face chats between medical experts and the public (Table 11.2). For example, a science popularization training range has been set up in the Shanghai Women and Children Service Guidance Center where thousands of people have benefited from the home care science popularization knowledge. In Xujiahui Huitai Business Mansion, "Da Yi Xiao Hu" established the first demonstration building for science popularization which held the "Let's get science popularization, Huitai!" seasonal activities continuously. This campaign delivered health thematic topics and benefited more than 1000 merchants.

"Da Yi Xiao Hu" science popularization team was launched at Guangdong Medical University as well as Centenarians Service Range in Suixi County, Guangdong Province. Up to now, the team has conducted more than 300 science popularization lectures and health counseling sessions which attracted more than 50,000 audiences.

1.4. *About talent training*

"Da Yi Xiao Hu" network studio and student group in Shanghai Jiao Tong University have been developed to find and train the science popularization talents among university students, especially in medical students. The team also attempts to set up a "Medical Communication" course in medical

Table 11.2 "Da Yi Xiao Hu" science popularization programs launched.

Code	Program	Person in charge
1	Yellow Bracelets — science popularization program for Alzheimer's disease in community	Jiang Ping
2	Establishing an evaluation and management system for bone health	Shi Huipeng
3	"Working Together to Save a Life" Cardiopulmonary Resuscitation Training Program	Zhou Minjie
4	"Let's get science popularization", Health science popularization for buildings	Ma Lulu
5	"Best Ayi" Home Care Standardization Program	Dai Qun
6	"Smart Blue-collar" Program	Shi Jiahua
7	On-campus Health Science Popularization Range	Zhu Jianhui
8	Star Doctor Lecturers' Group	Dai Hengwei
9	Da Yi Xiao Hu Student Group	Wang Qian
10	University Network Studio	Zhao Keyang
11	WeChat official account and official site operation and Maintenance	Yang Zhi
12	University electives: Medical Communication	Xu Zhongqing
13	"Laughter at ease" program	Zhao Jingke, Jiang Ping
14	Male Nurse Chorus	Fang Chenfei, Zhang Weiqing
15	Physician–Patient Relationship Research Studio	Wang Tao

schools and universities. "Da Yi Xiao Hu" has become the connotation construction project of Shanghai University think tank in 2018, which has been a new benchmark for university science popularization education and talent training.

1.5. *Science popularization research*

The team has obtained funding for a number of projects related to medical science popularization or medical communication research at provincial, ministerial, university, and health bureau levels. It has published several popular science research papers in core journals, such as Home Care for the Elder and Sick People in Community, Lifestyle Disease-Bone Health: Development and

Promotion of Spine and Joint Fitness Exercise Micro-Video by Shanghai Science and Technology Commission, and so on.

Collaborated with several institutions, the first "Framework Convention on Popular Health Science Dissemination" was launched in Zhanjiang.

"Da Yi Xiao Hu" jointly launched the first "Chinese Medical Communication Think Tank" with the 7th Medical Popular Science Committee of the China Science Writers Association, Popular Science Branch of the Chinese Medical Association, People's Daily Online, the Health Times, the China Online Health Channel, CN-Healthcare, and media. The elective course of medical communication has been launched in the School of Medicine, Shanghai Jiaotong University. "Teaching Demonstration Project of Medical Communication" has been founded in St Luke's Hospital affiliated to the Shanghai Jiaotong University School of Medicine where the team hosted a nationwide "Seminars on Medical Communication Teaching" aiming to generate new medical communication theory. The team also carried out a variety of academic seminars and science popularization forum, such as academic exchanges on the topics of "Da Yi Xiao Hu — Kidney and Heart" and "Da Yi Xiao Hu — Nutrition and Health".

2. Dissemination and community comments

The team has set up 92 online popular science columns with a total of nearly 600 original works to date. The posts had been viewed more than 100 million times annually and had benefited millions of people. It not only plays a great role in coaching the public for popular science, but also provides positive energy for the increasingly tense physician–patient relationship. The team focuses on shaping "Da Yi Xiao Hu" as an omnimedia brand of medical science popularization. In addition to running the "Da Yi Xiao Hu" official account to update daily all year round, it has also set up specific menus or columns on People's Daily Online, the China Online, Xinhua Net, Xinhua Daily Telegraph, Shanghai Xinmin Evening News, Chinese Science Communication, and Tencent Shanghai. Meanwhile, it has inducted into Shanghai News 163, Headlines Today, Tencent News,

Kuaibao, Particle News, Sina Weibo, Sohu, and CN-Healthcare. The posts had been viewed more than 200 million times and had been reposted by hundreds of media, which also featured on homepage of various portal websites. On April 11, 2017, "Da Yi Xiao Hu" signed a strategic coopera-tion framework agreement with People's Daily Online in Beijing. The team has also launched the "Da Yi Xiao Hu" popular science portal web-site which runs a salient home care program.

"Doctors and Nurses" and "Da Yi Xiao Hu" medical communication think tank have been branded "China Science Communication" by the Chinese Association of Science and Technology. It has won "Tencent Excellent People's Livelihood Account", "Tencent Best We Media Operating Award", First Prize in Shanghai Medical Association Youth Popular Science Competition, and "Top Ten News Events of Chinese Medical Popularization". In addition, the brand and its original works have also won the honors of outstanding achievements in medical ethics popularization in Shanghai, the Finalist in Jiangsu Public-Service Advertisements Competition, Honorable Mention in Popular Science Public-Service Advertisements Competition from Shandong Association for Science and Technology, Silver Award in "Healthy China, Beautiful Shanghai" Science Popular Public-Service Advertising Competition, Third Place Winner in Shanghai Medical System "Starlight Plan", Shanghai Science and Technology Achievement Award, and the "Best Director Award" in the Jury Prize of the 2017 Shanghai International Popular Science Micro Film Competition.

Teamwork has received dozens of publicity reports from mainstream media such as CCTV, People's Daily Online, Jie Fang Daily-Shanghai Observer, Wen Wei Po, Shanghai Xinmin Evening News, Health Times, Shanghai Science and Technology, Shanghai Television, and Shanghai Radio. The Chinese Medical Association, Shanghai Science and Technology Committee, Shanghai Association for Science and Technology, Chinese Science Writers Association jointly guided the "Da Yi Xiao Hu" academic seminar". On September 17, 2017, National Science Popularization Day, as a representative of the "Stay Healthy" project from Chinese Medical Association's, the team exhibited in Beijing and was inspected by Party and state leaders.

3. Development of "Da Yi Xiao Hu"

The development of "Da Yi Xiao Hu" has been through three phases.

3.1. *First phase*

On March 28, 2016, the WeChat official account of "Doctors and Nurses" was set up for medical science popularization. At the beginning, there were only three to five members in the team. The members conducted medical science popularization and run operation and maintenance of the official account in their spare time after busy clinical work. With the joining of passionate colleagues, the team has gradually grown in strength. The content of the official account has gradually completed the transformation from reproduction to original. All of the authors are first-line medical staffs or professionals with medical education background. On November 28, 2016, eight months after the establishment of the official account, China Association for Science and Technology officially included "Doctors and nurses" into the media matrix of China Science Communication. The official account was also authorized to use the brand logo of "China Science Communication".

3.2. *Second phase*

Nowadays, we are stepping into the era of "Everything is media". The science popularization team also rides the trend of the times. Based on the stable and mature operation of WeChat official account, the team has built the official website of "Da Yi Xiao Hu" and successively set up specific menus or columns on People's Daily Online, the China Online, Xinhua Daily Telegraph, Xinhua News app, Tencent Shanghai, Chinese Science Communication. Meanwhile, it has inducted into Healthy China platform of National Health Commission of the People's Republic of China, Shanghai News 163, Tencent News, Kuaibao, Headlines Today, Particle News, CN-Healthcare and Sohu. Thus, the team naturally completed the transformation from the WeChat official account only to "Da Yi Xiao Hu" omnimedia brand of medical science popularization.

3.3. *Third phase*

From the establishment of the WeChat official account to the upgrade of "Da Yi Xiao Hu" omnimedia medical science popularization brand, the team has experienced many major events, each of which was a landmark achievement. Since authorized by "China Science Communication" of China Association for Science and Technology, "Da Yi Xiao Hu" has gradually absorbed more than 200 medical and communication experts from 20 provinces and autonomous regions (including Xinjiang and Tibet) and has built 92 online columns and 20 launched programs. Besides, it also got the approval of "Shanghai University think tank connotation construction project". Step by step, "Da Yi Xiao Hu" again made a great change. Combined original works, we media operation, programs launch, talent training, and science popularization research together, "Da Yi Xiao Hu" medical communication think tank was founded.

Looking back at the journey, "Da Yi Xiao Hu" has gone through the transformation from a WeChat official account to an omnimedia platform, from reposting content from other writers or platforms to producing original works, from a group with just a few members to a professional team, from online communication to offline projects launched, from only written words to videos, comics, songs, and a variety of forms, from the local to the whole country, and from popular science practice to theoretical improvement. This is how academic popular science develops (Figure 11.1).

By the end of 2018, the "Da Yi Xiao Hu" team has obtained 32 various research projects at various levels, including National Social Science Fund Projects. The "Da Yi Xiao Hu" medical communication think tank was officially established. The think tank was awarded the brand of "China Science Popularization" by China Association for Science and Technology again in December 2018.

4. Summary

Viewed from a developmental perspective, the medical popularization WeChat official account "Doctors and Nurses" was created on March 28, 2016. It has taken only two years to set up more than 90 columns which disseminate medical knowledge all year round. The rapid development

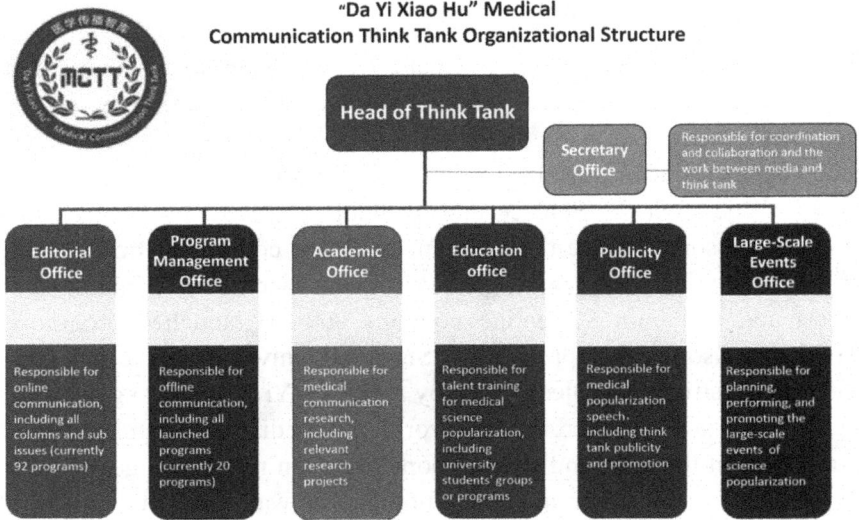

Figure 11.1 "Da Yi Xiao Hu" medical communication think tank organizational structure.

has also been welcomed by the public with total viewings at over 100 million annually.

Since the establishment of "Da Yi Xiao Hu", all the members of the team are clinical first-line medical staffs or professionals with medical education background. Medical communication and popularization must be carried out by professionals with medical knowledge, which is the principle of "Da Yi Xiao Hu". This can ensure the accuracy and reliability of medical knowledge to the fullest extent.

Since busy clinical work being doctors' daily routine, people would wonder whether they have time or mood to perform medical communication. Dr. Sun Simiao, a medical expert in the Tang Dynasty, wrote an article "Great Medical Ethics", in which he wrote, "Being doctors, they should regard patients' suffering as their own and have deep sympathy for them. Confronted with danger, they should not try to avoid it. No matter in the daytime or night, in winter or summer, and no matter when they are hungry or thirsty, tired or exhausted, they should work for the patients' heart and soul without any delay and contemplation for personal gain or loss. Only by doing so can one become a great doctor for the people. Otherwise he will surely become a scourge of the people." Yes, if a doctor can really "regard patients' suffering as their own", then it's understandable why they would contribute their spare time to support the medical science popularization, "no matter in the daytime or night, in winter or summer, and no matter when they are hungry or thirsty, tired or exhausted", aiming to achieve "no sickness, less sickness" for people. For medical staff, "help and cure people" is not only an occupation, but also a mission, and also the life itself.

It is evident from above that many medical professionals believe more efforts should be made to prevent the occurrence and development of diseases. This is also the reason that professionals are interested in and contribute their spare time to the medical communication and popularization. On the other hand, many medical professionals have realized that there are pseudoscience and pseudomedicine spread in the current medical science popularization. This makes medical professionals can't wait to make full use of their expertise and advantages to offer the medical knowledge properly. Furthermore, taking forward with the spirit of the "Great Medical Ethics", many medical professionals are willing to apply what they have learned to the public, not only in the treatment of diseases, but also in the popularization of the medical knowledge to the citizens. These are the important reasons why "Da Yi Xiao Hu" can quickly attract many medical professionals to participate.

In response to the large number of internet users in China, "Da Yi Xiao Hu" has used the advantages of new media and we media to spread medical knowledge on the internet since the establishment of the public account. At the beginning, it was relatively simple in content just with articles of medical science popularization in the WeChat official account. There are various forms gradually, including the medical comics "Yuanbei medical painting" and "Medical writing and painting", which are simple, beautiful, vivid and interesting medical illustrations and comics. Medical crosstalk column, "Education Goes Together with Pleasure", incorporates medical knowledge into crosstalk by "speaking, learning, teasing and singing". Similarly, "Laughter At Ease" popularizes medical knowledge to the audience. Videos also have been used for medical popularization, such as "80 Days Transformation". It is a team composed of one doctor and four male nurses to promote home care and family first aid guide using self-composed, self-directed, and self-acted videos. The guide is simple, easy to learn, and practical for home care and rehabilitation. Medical poetry column named as "Medical Journey With Poetry Spirit", shares all the joy of life with people; while medical music column, "Science Popularization Music" combines science popularization and music to make it more lively and interesting. It integrates theory and practice to explore popularization theory during music creation. The micro film column, "Science Education Film", cooperates with the Science and Educational Film Studio of Shanghai Film Group to bring the latest and best medical science films or documentaries which are from the senior producers and directors. There is a medical radio column, such as "Keep a Healthy Voice", which uses sound to improve people's mood, excite the feelings, and lift the spirits. Meanwhile, the "Listen to Health" reduces negative status including stress, anxiety, depression, and terror which are caused by social and psychological factors. This will improve the stress and pressure resistance ability of listeners and achieve the goal of "Listen to Health". With innovative forms, the above columns not only significantly enriched "Da Yi Xiao Hu"'s character, but also greatly broaden the audience population for medical communication because of the lively and interesting forms. Thus the influence of "Da Yi Xiao Hu" in the public has been gradually increased.

Discussing from the aspect of contents production, the columns of "Da Yi Xiao Hu" have achieved the practice of medical communication at three levels: about "disease", about "doctors visit", and about "perspectives on disease". Regarding the contents, most of the columns mainly focus on "disease", for example, "Pursuing Healthy Spine" and "Talk About Bone and Muscle". These columns include tertiary prevention, healthcare and wellness, rehabilitation, nursing, and child care education. "Health Insurance Notes" and "Tips for a Successful Doctor Visit" columns mainly focus on "doctors visit" that mostly provide guidance for how to make a successful doctor visit, as well as the legal knowledge related to healthcare and so on. "A Benevolent Mind and Excellent Skills", "Happiness Bank", and "Physician–Patient Relationship" are mainly discussions about "perspectives on disease" which guide people to understand and regard the disease properly. These columns help to make people understand the limitations of medicine and the importance of medical humanistic care. Sure, in terms of content, each column popularizes the medical knowledge from the various perspectives of the above three levels rather than limiting to a single level. However, the focus of each column is different.

In terms of medical communication channels, "Da Yi Xiao Hu" spreads medical knowledge not only through the new media and we media, but also launches many offline programs. For example, the health science popularization for Huitai Business Mansion has been carried out in the work place for white-collars who get the opportunities to learn medical knowledge. "Best Ayi" home care standardization training program is also one of the "Da Yi Xiao Hu" offline programs launched in the Shanghai Women and Children Service Guidance Center. A group of Ayi (domestic helpers) has been trained to have general medical and nursing knowledge and this has been warmly welcomed by the market.

In the development of "Da Yi Xiao Hu", there have been many achievements and praise. For example, the WeChat official account of "Da Yi Xiao Hu" won "Tencent Excellent People's Livelihood Account" and "Tencent Best We Media Operating Award". It was selected as "Top Ten News Events of Chinese Medical Popularization". The "Da Yi Xiao Hu" team joined the exhibition in Beijing on behalf of Chinese Medical Association on 2017 National Science Popularization Day. It also won the First Prize for Traditional Chinese Medical Science and Technology from Hunan Province and the third prize of Shanghai Medical Science and Technology Award. "Da Yi Xiao Hu" won the best organization award in the "New Era Health Science Popularization Works Collection" which was held by the National Health Commission, Ministry of Science and Technology, and China Association for Science and Technology. On October 25, 2018, the "Da Yi Xiao Hu" was invited to introduce "Experience of Health Promotion and Health Education" at the Press Conference held by the National Health Commission.

From the development process of "Da Yi Xiao Hu", it was clear that there is a growing demand for standardized medical science popularization. When reliable and accurate medical knowledge is popularized by medical professionals, it can be widely and effectively covered if we use various media and forms, including creative and novel ones, to make pedestrian versions for the public. Meanwhile, it can also promote the development of science popularization and medical communication.

Chapter 12

Medical Communication Scenarios in Different Contexts

Context refers to a situation that various conditions combined together or conflicted with each other in a certain period of time. It is also known as situation or circumstance. Context includes situation of play, given situation, teaching scenarios, social context, learning environment and so on. In social psychology, context also refers to the environmental condition that interferes with one's occurrence or behavior. In different contexts, the patterns, contents, and emphasis of medical communication can be different in some aspects. Some innovative forms can be involved as well.

1. Scenarios of communication in clinics

Various approaches are available for medical communication, of which the most classical one is communication in the clinic. Effective medical communication can be achieved at the time when patients are seeking help from clinicians: clinicians provide some points of medical communication in the process of diagnosis-making and treatment planning according to the situation and demand of each patient. The most common site for medical communication in clinics is the outpatient clinic, especially the specialist clinic. Clinicians have spare time to provide medical communication and health information for the patients because of their relatively mild illness; however, they are required to deal with the severe cases properly in a short period of time to help them out of danger. That is to say, size up

310

the situation before medical communication in emergency and always put every patient's life in the first place.

Here are some cases:

A patient visiting the specialist clinic presented with fever for three days, associated with a runny nose, nasal congestion, sore throat, and muscular soreness. He/she asked for antibiotic treatment as well as an intravenous infusion. A general impression of upper respiratory tract infection, commonly known as a cold, was diagnosed by the doctor according to a detailed medical history and physical examination. From a medical standpoint, there is no need for antibiotics or intravenous infusion in treatment of cold; however, the patient was difficult to understand it, as he/she thought they were necessary to relieve the fever and malaise. As for this patient, these useful ideas should be conveyed as the entry points for medical communication.

In fact, some harmful effects of intravenous infusion include adverse reaction, blockage in the vessels due to increasing number of insoluble particles, vulnerability to diseases, weakened immunity, and potential drug resistance. It is not recommended to apply intravenous infusion as a routine practice, unless necessary. Neither is antibiotic use. Antibiotics are primarily prescribed for bacterial infection, while common cold is mainly self-limiting viral infection; in other words, the patients may recover in several days without use of medications. But surely for those who combined with bacterial infection, antibiotics should be applied. Inappropriate use of antibiotics may lead to adverse outcomes, such as antibiotic resistance, and more seriously, so-called superbacteria resulting from abuse of antibiotics.

Intravenous infusion and antibiotics are effective treatments in people's minds. People don't know how they work, but they ask for them. It is firmly believed that these measures are able to cure diseases quicker. As a result, doctors should pay attention to the communication skills when they consider it unnecessary to prescribe antibiotics; otherwise, it doesn't work well if doctors refuse the patient's request clumsily. The establishment of trust and a harmonious communication atmosphere is a crucial footstone. Health education on antibiotics and intravenous infusion can be smoothly carried out during the guidance. It is helpful to use simple words and examples to communicate with the patients since they have little medical knowledge. Too many medical terms interfere with the effectiveness of communication, being difficult for patients to understand.

As clinicians are usually busy, the consulting time for each patient is generally restricted, which merely enables brief and straightforward communication. It would be better if waiting patients browse over the background information, which is prepared and placed around the clinic, with a combination of oral education by clinicians.

For example, several articles on harmful effects of intravenous infusion and antibiotics could be placed in the outpatient waiting area. Thus, more effectiveness can be achieved in less time when clinicians give them oral education in line with their actual situations.

2. Cases of communication in community and public occasions

A community is a body of persons or social organizations of common and especially professional interests correlated with each other and scattered through a larger society, with certain interaction and maintenance of common culture. It is widely believed that constitutive elements of community are a certain number of people, certain range of territory, certain scale of facilities, certain characteristics of culture, and certain types of organizations. Community is such a social group of people who inhabit a special region.

A community generally has the following features: within a special geographical area, a certain number of people, common awareness and interests among residents and close social contact.

Medical communication in community, as the name suggests, is the popularization and communication of medical knowledge in the community. The contents should be relative to the residents and those they concern about, according to the meaning and features of a community. Let's talk about some examples.

Open occasions, such as communities and public places, are suitable for larger and more interactive educational communication activities, in which more people will take part, compared with one-to-one communication in clinics.

There are two types of medical communication in community. Firstly, the one aimed at a particular group with a specific topic. For example, medical workers provide communication and popularization on the prevention of myopia for primary and secondary schools. Secondly, the one without fixed population. For instance, education on prevention of hypertension held by medical workers in the hospital hall. Every patient or their relatives who come to the hospital on that day can participate in the communication if they like.

For a specific population, the first step is to understand their health problems or demands. Then set out the content, when, where, and how to do it.

For example, if the employees are mostly young, especially female employees of child-bearing age, they need more knowledge on maternal and infant care. Medical workers can provide knowledge on breastfeeding and vaccination through the communication. The effect may not be good enough if the content is chosen irrelevantly.

Let's take the "yellow bracelet" in AD prevention as an example of medical communication in a community.

Alzheimer's disease (AD) is an insidious-onset, progressive neurodegenerative disease of unknown etiology, with dysmnesia, aphasia, apraxia, agnosia, visuospatial dysfunction, executive dysfunction, personality, and behavioral change as the clinical manifestation. An onset age of younger than 65 is called presenile dementia, while an onset age of older than 65 is defined as senile dementia.

The quality of life worsens severely once one gets AD. The most common symptom is memory loss. The patients become easy to forget things even if they try hard to remember and they are unable to recall them afterwards, which interferes with their daily activities seriously. With further development of the disease, the patients suffer from inability in dressing, eating, urination and defecation. They can't recognize their spouse and children. Some may present with hallucinations. Endless misery is brought about to the patients themselves and their relatives as their activities of daily living (ADL) decrease inevitably. The mean survival time of AD patients is 6 years. It is not those who have AD that suffer most, but those who take care of them. Among all the relatives who look after AD patients, more than 80 percent of them have mood disorder of different degrees. Some of them even suffer from depression and anxiety disorder. It is not only the fatigue, but also the hopelessness and inability to communicate that makes them feel desperate. A 10-year cost of 400,000 RMB for an AD patient is estimated, excluding daily cost of living and food, which is equivalent to a well-located house in a second-tier city.

By 2020, there will be at least 150,000 families in Shanghai faced with AD patients and their caring responsibility. Thus, it is both a social and medical problem for Shanghai to deal with urgently to popularize relevant knowledge of AD in all society and cope with the challenge of an aging society. It is of great significance to hold activity to popularize scientific knowledge on AD to community residents and the elder population. The "yellow bracelet" project relies on Tangqiao community in Pudong district to carry out a variety of scientific activities about AD among the residents, which aims at the conflict between explosion of AD patients as a result of aging society and lack of AD knowledge in citizens. As the proverb goes, give a man a fish and you feed him for a day; teach a man to fish and you feed him for a lifetime. Hopefully, the following objectives can be met through this scientific educational activity in the community. First, provide AD knowledge and the dilemma AD patients faced with for residents, including lack of social support, professional care for AD patients, protection of legitimate rights, and interests of patients. Then provide the patients and their carers with relevant guidance and support on medical, caring, and living aspect to help improve their quality of life and enjoy their later years. Secondly, call on all walks of life to know AD, care for AD patients and their family members, work together to establish a community culture, pay attention to the yellow bracelet, and care for the elderly. Finally, the formation of a social custom that all society care about the mental health of elderly and the elderly care for their health behaviors and quality of life contribute to a harmonious society.

The team did an investigation of the Tangqiao community before they carried out the project. The investigation reveals a highly aging Tangqiao community with more than 22% of the elderly aged 60 or more in the permanent resident population. AD has been a significant health problem that severely threatens the residents. It not only brings a heavy financial and mental burden to the family, but also creates tremendous pressure on the society. The implementation of "yellow bracelet" project meets with the actual demand of inhabitants in Tangqiao as well as the construction plan of "healthy and supportive community" in the next round of development.

According to the above investigation, the project team cooperated with home fitness community service. Many specialists in prevention and treatment of AD from several tertiary hospitals, like Shanghai Mental Health Center (SMHC), were invited to share a series of scientific feasts in prevention and treatment of AD with the residents, which aimed at enhancing their awareness of AD prevention and offering help to their family so as to promote the entire capability of AD prevention and treatment.

On August 24, 2016, the opening ceremony of scientific exhibition and the launch of 'yellow bracelet' activity in Tangqiao community was held on the stage of cultural activity center of Tangqiao in Pudong district, which was an official sign of the beginning of a scientific series of activities.

The activities were full of variety and forms. Professional scientific education of AD was provided from multiple dimensions, such as prevention, diagnosis, treatment, home nursing, and psychological counseling. Over 500 audiences were attracted by 6 exhibitions held from August 2016 to December 2016. Four specific lectures on AD containing early identification and intervention of AD, home caring for AD patients and mental nursing for both patients and relatives were conducted, which covered more than 300 residents. Two hundred residents were organized to watch the documentary film *Please Remember Me*, a film that reflects the life of AD patients, on September 21, 2016, the world Alzheimer's day. A science carnival was held before the Christmas in 2016. Multiple health counseling and services were offered: health consultation of cognitive dysfunction, mental health, Traditional Chinese Medicine, general practice and neurology from different hospitals, examination tests such as blood pressure, blood sugar, and bone mineral density, and policy consulting services as well. Through the health service for AD prevention and treatment provided in the doorway, the health demand was fulfilled with an enhanced health awareness and improved ability to self-care and prevent AD. In addition, seven interactive fun games were organized with over 300 participants. Each family was given a brochure and a popular science book, with a total of over 200 families.

The scientific activities were reported by seven media for ten times in six months, which communicated with the society about the current situation of AD population and knowledge on AD to the greatest extent. Two TV channels, two newspapers, two official accounts, and one network were included.

As the online platform of this science popularization activity, "Yellow Bracelet Home", relying on WeChat public account, the fastest transmission way in the era of mobile Internet, has assisted the series of science popularization activities to advance step by step and enhance the participation of community residents. In addition, the project was also publicized on the largest all-media medical science popularization platform "Da Yi Xiao Hu" in China. After various media reports, the project has made contributions to the formation of the culture of respecting the elderly, caring for the mental health of the elderly, caring for their own health behavior, and quality of life.

A brand new form of scientific popularization is invented domestically: popularization of science through comic dialogue. It was really surprising to the residents that two beautiful girls performed comic dialogue during the carnival in December 2016. This was the first time they enjoyed popularization of science through comic dialogue and comic dialogue by two girls. The program was "dotard", a story describing an old man with various mistakes that result from AD. It was well-designed and the residents couldn't help laughing. Two key points are popularized to the population in a joyful atmosphere: first, the cognitive function of AD patients is gradually decreasing; secondly, enough patience is necessary for the relatives to take care of the patients. Much laughter and happiness were brought about by the team from crosstalk association of Shanghai Jiao Tong University School of Medicine. The team consists of several clinical professionals who produce and perform the play. They focus on crosstalk about medical science and devote themselves to translation of professional medical knowledge to language arts by means of crosstalk, which enables the audience to learn about medical knowledge through happiness and cheerful laughter. In the future, a joint effort will be made with the crosstalk team to explore more innovative models of science popularization and educational activities in the community, to provide genuine welfare for our residents.

The project team uploaded the above-mentioned contents to the Cloud, including a 7-minute science popularization film (798M, MPG), six AD relevant activities in a series of yellow bracelet campaign and two articles published on the official account "yellow bracelet home" sharing some inspiration from off-line events. With the implementation and communication of the "yellow bracelet" project in Tangqiao community, the medical knowledge of AD in local residents has been increased markedly.

For medical communication without fixed population, the topics should fit for the majority of people rather than those with distinct geographical or population characteristics. If a seminar on cerebral infarction is held in a maternal and child health hospital, there will be few audience because the majority population is women and children who are not at high risk for cerebral infarction and they have no such concerns. That is why there would be few participants and poor effect even if the activity is held. However, the same situation in an integrated hospital or an aging community will be effective and appealing to lots of elderly people and those who have cerebral infarction. Similarly, the participants will shoot up if a specific lecture on pregnancy and child-rearing knowledge is conducted in the maternal and child health hospital.

Interaction is of great importance when many participants are involved in the communication. If the lecturer merely repeats what the book says, listeners are usually sleepy even if the lecturer puts great effort into it. Vivid factors, such as crosstalk and play, can be added to the lesson to get the audience involved in. Prize-giving quiz can be put into practice and questions in accord with personal situation are welcomed. Involvement of both sides is more effective than unilateral instilled education.

3. Medical communication in work place

Most of us have our jobs in various work places or offices. Work places are where workers do their daily work. For instance, the streets and roads are work places of sanitation workers. Offices are work places for white-collar workers and supermarkets are those for supermarket assistants.

Some other explanations include places where we can learn, develop one's potential and personality, obtain living expenses, interact, and compete with others.

Medical communication in work places is convenient for workers there. At the same time, the contents should be selected properly to maximize the effectiveness according to their distribution and interests.

Let's have a look at the communication in Huitai building in Shanghai.

This building (previously power building) is an office building for rent, with convenient transportation links, located in a prosperous commercial developmental zone on Xujiahui Road in Huangpu district, and is attached to Shanghai Electricity Industrial Corporation. It is divided into a 23-storey main building and a 9-storey annex building, with a total area of 26,189 square meters, over 1000 office workers and nearly 30 tenants.

On February 17, 2017, the joint project by "Da Yi Xiao Hu" started at Huitai building. It was the first demonstration building by "Da Yi Xiao Hu" and the committee of medical health in science popularization writer association in Shanghai; this opened a new model of science popularization in buildings. On the same day, an activity with the theme of prevention and treatment of cold at the end of winter and the beginning of spring was held. Thirty tenants and owners took part in the interaction, which was an attempt of health culture in new types of buildings and a concrete practice of the layout plan *Healthy China 2030*.

Dr. Chen from Shanghai Children's Medical Center (SCMC) established an information desk in Huitai building for those white-collars in his leisure time at the noon of July 7, 2017. The theme was "classroom for parents" in summer vacation. In total 40 parents were received per hour, which was equivalent to the half-day outpatient visits in SCMC.

It was greatly appreciated by the white-collars that they can have specialist counseling in the company after lunch. Some came in with similar troubles. A couple working in the same building came to complain about the daily living issues of their twins coincidently.

One of the parents commented that there would not be enough time to communicate with clinicians face to face if he visited a specialist clinic in the hospital. The one-hour experience brought about a different feeling to Dr. Chen as well: both the patients and the doctor were more relaxed and straightforward, like chatting among friends.

This was the first attempt of Huitai building. A two-month cultural season of science popularization was held in Huitai building in 2017, witnessed by municipal science and technology committee, association for science and technology, experts on science popularization and media. Eight sessions were carried out, from maintenance of shoulder and neck and moxa-moxibustion to healthy concept of life and psychological relief, which perfectly fit the demands of white-collar workers, making it possible for them to receive health information indoors.

Meanwhile, an online survey was delivered to hundreds of white-collar workers in Huitai building to acquire their demands for information about science popularization. Via two months of data collection and statistical analysis, it revealed that nearly 70% of the white-collar workers were quite interested in children's health, maintenance of cervical spine, physical therapy, and mental health. Specific to the realistic needs of the workers, elaborately designed second season lit up the summer and autumn of Huitai building. Seven sessions were more suitable and precise, which were warmly welcomed and highly recognized. Along with the solid foundation, the project actively fed the media with information to expand the social effect and influence of science popularization, which is reported by mainstream media like Shanghai Evening Post and Wen Hui Bao. The project brand is successfully created.

Compared with traditional science popularization lectures, those in work places enable the workers to participate in some scientific activities that they are interested in. They can acquire the knowledge they need using leisure time without going far. Undoubtedly, good effects can be achieved only when the contents of medical communication and science popularization in work places are related to the workers' need. If the local workers are mainly unmarried youth, then it is not effective enough to provide communication in child rearing.

The following specialties should be made to attract more audiences and strengthen the effect. First of all, a superior topic is the key determinant of whether the audiences can be gained. Precision is reflected by the learning points. The lessons are given as the audiences ask for. Care is reflected through services that realize the full coverage of service information in building, making the health knowledge at fingertips. Mutual benefits reflect the sincerity of cooperation to ensure its living space and help brand promotion. The stance is to fulfill the national strategy of realizing the comprehensive health of the entire people throughout life. The concerns are focused on functional community so that the marginal group can enjoy health information at ease. Secondly, emotional interaction is of great importance. It can be achieved by means of close contact and emotion investment regardless of the forms. It can only be a product for self-entertainment if the lecture stays at a form of preaching. The audience will be triggered to participate with passion through empathy if the lecturer puts much effort into the lecture, making it true to life. Emotion is always the indispensable core and the common language to connect to all levels of audiences as a whole. The lecturer should express his/her care about the health of the audience. Thirdly, the pattern of manifestation determines whether the audience will be kept or not. We encourage a vigorous form and reject depression. A simple soul can be decorated with beautiful packaging full of new media elements. Medical science popularization should pay attention to current trends to make it popular. The brand is supposed to be pleasant to hear, easy to remember, useful, and interesting.

Chapter 13

Exploration of Innovative Medical Communication

Innovation is the behavior that improves or creates new inventions, methods, elements, paths, environments, and abilities, gaining positive effects with the existing knowledge and resources. Innovation in line with the idealized needs or the need of society, is guided by but different from conventional or ordinary ideas. Innovation is a unique cognitive ability and practical ability of human, also the advanced expression of subjective initiative, and the inexhaustible motive force to promote national progress and social development. If a country wants to lead the world, it couldn't stop the innovation and innovative thinking for a moment. Innovation plays an important role in the fields of economy, technology, sociology, and architecture. In essence, innovation is the externalization, materialization, and formalization of the innovative thinking.

With the rapid development of modern technology, innovative forms are needed to speed up the popularization of medical communication and to strengthen its effect.

The science popularization of health is to popularize the healthy lifestyle in public, to acknowledge the public to establish health consciousness and to develop good living behaviors. Nowadays in an omnimedia age, innovative forms of science popularization in modernized and easy-to-understand language are necessary.

1. Cases of new media and We Media communication

New media is an environment in which everyone becomes the media. In short, new media is an environment.

New media is a kind of media form with the support of new technology systems, including digital magazine, digital newspaper, digital radio, short message, mobile TV, network, desktop window, digital TV, digital movie, and touch media. Compared to the four traditional media forms such as newspaper, outdoor media, radio, and television, new media is vividly called as "the fifth media".

New media is a broad definition. It provides users the information and the entertainment service on the terminals of computer, mobile phone and digital television with digital technology and network technology in the channels of internet, the broadband local network, the wireless network, the satellite, and others. Strictly speaking, new media should be called as "digital new media".

Nowadays, there are many new forms of new media such as WeChat, Weibo, Post Bar, Tik Tok, and so on. Researchers found that it took 38 years for radio to spread to 50 million people; for television 13 years, for the internet 4 years, and for Weibo only 14 months, which shows the fast development of new media. It is no doubt that the use of new media for medical communication will have an extraordinary effect.

Many medical institutions, including medical association, association of physicians, and major hospitals have realized the importance of new media. They set up official accounts on WeChat and Weibo to spread and communicate medical knowledge. The best advantages of new media lie in timeliness and regional popularity. For example, at the winter and spring alternated time of last year, the flu broke out in various regions of our country. Some major new media began to publicize and popularize knowledge on flu. On the one hand, it effectively met the needs of the public in time. On the other hand, as long as there is a mobile phone and network, people can receive the information from new media, which has full coverage in each area. This is another effect that cannot be achieved by office transmission or other media.

We Media, also called "civic media" or "personal media", refers to private, civilian, general, autonomous communicators. We Media communicates normative and non-normative information to unspecified majority or specific individuals in modern and electronic ways. We Media platforms include Blog, Weibo, WeChat, Baidu official Post Bar, forum/BBS, and other network communities.

In July 2003, the Media Center of American Press Society announced a report of "We Media", co-sponsored by Sheynkman and Chris Willis, in which there is a very strict definition of "We Media". We Media is a way to understand how ordinary people provide and share their own facts and news after being strengthened through digital technology and by the general public connected to the global knowledge system. In short, We Media is the carrier used by citizens to publish events they have seen and heard, such as Blog, Weibo, WeChat, forum/BBS, and other network communities.

Many specialists or ordinary medical staff have their WeChat accounts to spread medical knowledge, which can be seen as a form of medical communication by We Media. For example, Dr. Duan Tao, former president of Shanghai First Maternal and Infant Health Institute, has his personal WeChat official account "Dr. Duan Tao", with which he often spreads and popularizes medical knowledge about maternal and children health, such as "Which is the best oral administration contraceptive medicine?", "Why is it important for pregnant women to control blood sugar on pregnancy?" Each article attracts ten thousand readers.

The medical science popularization brand, "Da Yi Xiao Hu" introduced in the earlier chapter is a brand of science popularization of medicine for public welfare, integrating talent training, original works, self-media operation, entity building, science popularization, and science popularization academic research. It owns various We Media platforms including WeChat account "Da Yi Xiao Hu", which is operated by the medical staff in spare time, as an authoritative, scientific, objective, and public welfare medical science popularization platform, and carries out continual medical communication online every day in all medical fields.

2. Talk shows in the science popularization of health and medical knowledge

The creation and spread of talk shows in the science popularization of health and medical knowledge in the community and online is a practical exploration of innovative medical communication forms.

With the experience of long time, the team called "Da Yi Xiao Hu — Laughter Is the Best Medicine" firstly established a new form, medical science talk show, as the form in popularization of health and medical knowledge in China. Editing medical and health knowledge into talk shows, and popularizing health knowledge to the public in laughter shows the perfect combination with medical knowledge and talk show.

Talk show is a folk performance art which originated from daily life and is popular among the masses. It learns extensively on the skills of other arts, such as oral art, storytelling and others during its development. Talk shows often use ironic language to show the true, the good, and the beautiful, and making people laugh is one of talk show's artistic features, with "speaking, imitating, teasing, and singing" as the main forms of expression. There are three types of talk show: in single, in pair, and in group. A talk show in single is performed by a single actor telling jokes. A talk show in pair is performed by two actors, between whom usually one is to amuse the audience, another is to bring out the comedy atmosphere. A talk show in group is performed by more than two actors. The traditional talk shows mainly satirize various old facts in the old society and reflect various phenomena in life with humorous narratives. Nowadays, in addition to carrying forward traditions, talk shows also praise new people and new things.

Talk show actors don't perform like narrators and storytellers or other performers do, nor perform like the actors in theater plays, they mainly perform as interlocutors. The lines of the talk show are not narrative, but dialogue (question and answer), which is more apparent in the kind of so-called "Mom–Son" talk show. In fact, in another kind of talk show called "Yi-Tou-Chen", the actor who is to amuse the audience and another actor who is to bring out the comedy atmosphere are also engaged in dialogue. Although the former's lines have some narrative in the content, it is still in the form of a dialogue between the actors. Here, the narrative in the lines is only spoken as an answer in dialogue, but cannot be told separately from the dialogue background. It is well known that talk show is an art which is good at communicating with audiences. The comedic effect in theater produced by talk shows is better than by the others. In addition to the reason for comedic effect in content, the form of dialogue in talk show, as a unique artistic expression, is another important reason for its popularization. In narrative art, the creators are confident that they have the power to seize the "inner essence" from several isolated events, and give the events the order of causal connections to form the fictional plot and communicate these contents with the audience. Therefore, the spread of information in talk show is basically one-way, and the audience passively accept the information.

In previous talk show performances, there are several different schools. A talk show in pair or in group is performed by two or more than two actors, in whom usually one is to amuse the audience called "Dou Gen", another is to bring out the comedy atmosphere called "Peng Gen". The actor "Dou Gen" mainly tells the storyline when performing and is now usually referred to as "A". The actor "Peng Gen" is an actor who narrates the storyline with "Dou Gen" during the performance and is now usually referred to as "B". In the talk show, the actor "Peng Gen" and the actor "Dou Gen" cooperate with each other through the setting up of story, gradually making up the story in the narration, and producing jokes. There are some actors good at being "Dou Gen" such as Mr. Ma (Ma Sanli), Mr. Hou (Hou Baolin), Mr. Chang (Chang Baoyu), Mr. Su (Su Wenmao), Mr. Ma (Ma Ji). There are some actors good at being "Peng Gen" such as Mr. Li (Li Wenhua), Mr. Tang (Tang JieZhong), Mr. Zhao (Zhao ShiZhong). These different kinds of talk shows are slightly different in performance content and form. However, there have been no talk shows mainly performed by medical staff, and few talk shows in medical science.

The team "Da Yi Xiao Hu — Laughter Is the Best Medicine" specializes in the creation and performance of medical science talk shows. Firstly, professional medical staff create medical science talk shows to ensure the content is scientific and professional. Secondly, talk show is selected as a popular art form, which ensures both artistic and fun features of the popularization. The research team of "Da Yi Xiao Hu — Laughter Is the Best Medicine" owns the copyright and performance rights of these creative works.

The goal of the team "Da Yi Xiao Hu — Laughter Is the Best Medicine" is to create talk shows in medical science, an innovative form of popular science in health education in China for the first time, to create/perform a series of medical science talk shows for residents in Shanghai, and to promote the talk show in all media (online and offline). The team spreads medical science talk shows, and explores the application of talk shows in the popularization of health and medical knowledge in omnimedia.

The team creates a series of talk shows in medical science which are divided into two categories: (1) Helping healthy residents correct risk factors such as bad living habits and unhealthy behaviors, improve self-care knowledge awareness and ability, and reduce the morbidity — "Prevention". (2) Most of the aged and patients with chronic diseases mainly rely on home care. With the talk show in medical science, the caregivers improve the scientific care ability, and then guide patients to consciously follow the doctor's instructions, to use medications properly, to choose a reasonable diet and appropriate exercise methods, and to promote the recovery of the disease earlier — "Treatment".

In addition to performing in the community, the promotion online of talk show in medical science was completed in the science popular omnimedia brand "Da Yi Xiao Hu" (online), which is a brand of medical science popularization in public welfare, and integrates talent training, original works, self-media operation, offline base building, science popularization, and science popularization academic research. At present, the number of page view is more than 100 million per year. In addition to cooperating with the WeChat public account of "Da Yi Xiao Hu", it also runs on columns in the People's Net, "Science Popular Cloud", Tencent Dashen.com, Xinhua Daily Telegraph, Xinhua News app, Xinmin Evening Newspaper, Today's Headline, Yidian News, Tencent News app, Daily Express, Netease Shanghai and other media with more than 30 million readers. It creates and performs original talk shows in medical science (offline) for residents in community, and promotes the talk shows in "Da Yi Xiao Hu" online. The team fully explores the establishment and the application of the medical science talk show in the popularization of health and medical knowledge with omnimedia.

As 2016 to 2017, the team created and performed five talk shows, including "Old Mess" on December 22, 2016; "Bicycle Sharing" on May 31, 2017; "Smoking Hobby" on May 31, 2017; "I Don't Know" on September 21, 2017; "Amnesia" on September 21, 2017.

As the launch of above five original talk shows in medical science has received enthusiastic response from the audience, foreign friends hope to join in science popularization activities in China. On September 21, 2017, the first attempt was made by foreign volunteers to participate in a talk show in medical science. In 2018, a team named "Cheerful Science Popularization" focusing on the medical science talk show with foreign science popularization volunteers was set up.

The performances of the team "Cheerful Science Popularization" in medical science talk show are shown in Table 13.1.

Its aim is to develop "Cheerful Science Popularization" into another innovative popular science form both offline and online, that is distinctive, systematic, sustainable, influential, and welcomed, spreading health knowledge in public in laughter.

It is a platform for foreign friends to communicate with science popularization in China, and to explore the "Chinese model" of international science popularization. Now there are six foreign science popularization volunteers from six countries working in the activities, which has brought an extraordinary spreading effect.

Nowadays, the government strongly advocates the establishment of a lifelong learning society, and the public has become the targeted audience of science popularization service. Medical science popularization activities should match the needs of the people, serve the people, benefit the people, and carry out science popularization activities in keeping with the needs of the people. But no matter facing any object, communicators should always jump out of the old way and create innovative popular science form and content to attract more people.

Table 13.1 The performances of the team "Cheerful Science Popularization".

Number	Time	Title	Volunteer	Nationality	Performance	Spread online	Type
1	20170921	Amnesia	Максим	Russia	Tangqiao Community Center	Weibo	One Episode of talk show in medical science
2	20180125	Basic introduction	Andrew Fralick	America	Tangqiao Community Center	CHTV Weibo	One Episode of Talk show in medical science
3	20180411 20180724	Lady of Bone	Gufran	Turkey	No.2 PingNan Community Center Gulonghui Community Center	Weibo	Multiple episodes of talk show in medical science
4	20180828	Orthopedic specialist	Mi Mi Khaing	Myanmar	Gulonghui Community Center	Weibo	
5	20180920	Orthopedic diseases	Moawez Awan	Pakistan	Gulonghui Community Center	Weibo	
6	20181129	Risk of orthopedic diseases	Dilshat Pernebek Mi Mi Khaing	Kazakhstan Myanmar	Gulonghui Community Center	Miaopai Weibo	
7	20181213	Risk of orthopedic diseases for female	Moawez Awan	Pakistan	Gulonghui Community Center	Weibo	
8	20190118	Young with healthy bones	Moawez Awan	Pakistan	Gulonghui Community Center	Weibo	
Total	Eight original talk shows		Six foreign science popularization volunteers from six countries		Nine performances in communities. With more than 1800 audiences	More than 610 thousands audiences online	

Note: The medical science talk show is an innovative form of medical science popularization in China. "Cheerful Science Popularization" focuses on medical science talk shows with foreign science popularization volunteers.

The community is progressing, and the demands of the public are increasing. If we only use the out-of-date ideas to carry out medical science popularization, it will not bring better communication effects. Innovation should be used to grasp the needs and concerns of the public with a better communication effect. The medical science talk shows and "Cheerful Science Popularization" undoubtedly are good and popular attempts in this field.

www.ingramcontent.com/pod-product-compliance
Lightning Source LLC
Chambersburg PA
CBHW050539190326
41458CB00007B/1835